HAIR ADDITIONS
THE FOURTH DIMENSION

DEDICATED TO
Professional hairstylists
who never stop learning!

HAIR ADDITIONS
THE FOURTH DIMENSION

CHARLOTTE JAYNE

> Milady Publishing Company acknowledges that the printing process employed did not result in an accurate representation of the fine quality original color slides submitted by the author. Future printings will be of a much higher quality.

Milady Publishing Company
(A Division of Delmar Publishers Inc.)
220 White Plains Road, Tarrytown, New York 10591

Editor:	Catherine Frangie
Photographer:	Chuck Montague
Illustrators:	Marcie Gonzalez
	Stephanie Schultz

Copyright © 1991
Milady Publishing Company
(A Division of Delmar Publishers Inc.)

All rights reserved. No part of this work covered by the copyright hereon may be reproduced in any form or by any means—graphic, electronic, or mechanical, including photocopying, recording, taping, or information storage and retrieval systems--without written permission of the publisher.

Printed in the United States of America

10 9 8 7 6 5 4 3 2 1

Library of Congress Cataloging-in-Publication Data

Jayne, Charlotte, 1939-
  Hair additions: the fourth dimension/Charlotte Jayne.
    p.   cm.
  Includes index.
  ISBN 0-87350-390-2
  1. Hairweaving.   I. Title.
TT975.J39   1991   91-6337
646.7'245--dc20   CIP

TABLE of CONTENTS

PREFACE . . . . *ix*

ACKNOWLEDGMENTS . . . . *xi*

Chapter 1 **INTRODUCTION** 1
   What Is Your Business? 1
   What Is The Fourth Dimension? 2
   What This Book Is About 3
   Who Wants/Needs Hair Addition Services? 3
   Hair Has No Sex – Hair Has No Race! 4
   Why Now? 6
   Why and How It Affects the Industry 7
   Definition of Terms 8
   Information about Human Hair 11
   Information about Synthetic Fibers 19
   Attachment Techniques 20
   Summary 23

Chapter 2 **BRAIDING AND SEWING TRACKS** 25
   Introduction 25
   Advantages and Disadvantages 26
   Supplies 26
   Exercises 28
   Manikin Set Up 35
   Under Braid 35
   Under Filler Fiber Braid 42
   Under Braid on Scalp 51
   Under Filler Fiber Braid on Scalp 60
   Making Braided Tracks 70
   Finishing off Tracks 81
   Attaching Wefts to Tracks 83
   Maintaining and Re-Doing the Style 88
   Summary 88

Chapter 3 **INDIVIDUAL BRAIDING TECHNIQUES** 89
   Introduction 89
   Advantages and Disadvantages 90
   Supplies 91
   Speed-Bonding Technique 91
   Braid-in Tie-off with Loose Hair Technique 110
   Braid-in Tie-off with Thread Technique 122
   Separate Tie-off Technique 123
   Determining Hair Density and Placement 124
   Maintaining and Re-Doing the Style 125
   Summary 126

Chapter 4 BONDING TECHNIQUES ... 127
Introduction ... 127
Advantages and Disadvantages ... 128
Supplies ... 129
Attaching Wefts ... 129
Maintaining and Re-Doing the Style ... 133
General Comments ... 135
Summary ... 136

Chapter 5 PERMING FOR HAIR EXTENSIONS ... 137
Introduction ... 137
Supplies ... 138
Facts to Know about Wefts ... 138
Pre-Perm Analysis ... 140
Selecting the Perm Products ... 142
Wrapping Techniques ... 143
How to Perm Wefts ... 143
Becoming an Expert ... 149
Summary ... 150

Chapter 6 COLORING FOR HAIR EXTENSIONS ... 151
Introduction ... 151
Supplies ... 152
Facts to Know about Wefts ... 152
Pre-Color Analysis ... 155
About Color Products ... 155
The Rules – The Law of Color ... 156
How to Color Wefts ... 158
Becoming an Expert ... 161
Summary ... 162

Chapter 7 DESIGNING AND STYLING TECHNIQUES ... 163
Introduction ... 163
Supplies ... 163
Design Variations ... 164
    Introduction ... 164
    Basic Two-Tracks ... 164
    Basic Three-Tracks ... 165
    Full Coverage Six-Tracks ... 166
    Circular Four-Tracks ... 167
    Circular for Complete Coverage ... 168
    Brush-Back/Brush-Up ... 169
    Fashion Fun – Ponytail ... 169
    Fashion Fun – Asymmetrical ... 170
    Fashion Fun – Bangs ... 170
    Fashion Fun – Volume ... 170

TABLE OF CONTENTS

      Fashion Fun – Color Accents 171
      Combinations 172
   Cutting the Style 172
   Curling/Finishing 174
   Summary 174

Chapter 8 **PUTTING IT ALL TOGETHER** 175
   Introduction 175
   Supplies 179
   Consultation Objectives 180
   Consultation Work Sheet 181
      Introduction: 181
        1. Reason for Extensions: 183
        2. Life Style: 183
        3. Home Care Habits: 183
        4. Salon Habits: 184
        5. Stature: 184
        6. Hair Condition: 184
        7. Hair Texture: 184
        8. Hair Porosity: 184
        9. Hair Elasticity: 185
       10. Hair Density: 185
       11. Hair Form: 185
       12. Scalp Condition: 185
       13. Hair Length: 185
       14. Desired Length: 185
       15. Hair Color: 186
       16. Sensitive To: 186
       17. Growth Patterns: 186
       18. Facial Shape: 188
       19. Shape of Head: 189
      Placement Pattern 190
      Pricing Work Sheet 192
   Sample Services Price Sheet 195
   Hair Costing Sheet 196
   Hair Pricing Sheet 198
   Chemical Services Release Statement 199
   Hair Extension Agreement 200
   Model's Release 202
   Hair Extension Release Form 203
   Chemical Service Record 204
   Home Care Instruction Sheet 205
   Summary 210

Chapter 9 **CASE STUDIES** 211
   Introduction 211

Monnique	214
Dana	216
Leann	218
Larry	220
Wanda	222
Zettoria	224
Arlene	226
Marla	228
Ramin	230
Jennifer	232
Alondra	234
Candida	236
Janice	238
Susan	240
Lynn	242
Kathleen	244
Erin	246
General Comments	248
Chapter 10 **SALES AND MARKETING**	249
Introduction	249
Advertising	249
Public Relations	249
Sample News Release	250
Sample Editorial	251
Sample Letter to Editor	252
Community Activities	253
In-Salon Sales	253
A New Life -- A New Dimension	254
INDEX	255

PREFACE

This book is dedicated to the professional stylist who never stops learning – because learning is part of an active life.

As Dr. Eden Ryl, an expert in human behavior, discusses in the film *The Joy of Involvement*, "I think there are a lot of things we do every day that we really don't realize how little we know ... just simple tasks or assignments that we take on and don't understand what we're doing or why we're doing it. And when we do understand it takes on a whole new meaning."

Where Are You?

Behavior indicates involvement or non-involvement. Use the double helix (pictured right) to identify your feelings. Remember, world-famous musicians practice scales and finger exercises every day. Championship golfers constantly work at improving their swing and their putting. Ballet dancers never let a day go by without exercising. There is **no** task, however simple, mundane or routine that cannot be done better!

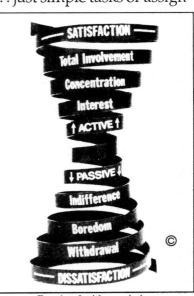

Reprinted with permission from The Joy of Involvement *a Ramic Productions film starring Dr. Eden Ryl.*

Graduating from school and receiving your license is *just the beginning*. You have been given only the basic tools, the basic knowledge with which to begin. Maybe, we ought to call our business the *practice* of cosmetology, as medical doctors have a practice in medicine.

With your license, you now have permission to begin your life in our industry. *The rest is up to you*. It is practice, setting a goal of doing your best, challenging yourself – that will bring you a life and a career of total involvement, of satisfaction and fulfillment.

Whether you are still a student or you have been practicing for 30 years – this book is written for those of you who want to reach out, for those of you who want to be totally involved.

As you work through this book I hope you will remember this statement by Dr. Ryl; "... there are a lot of things we do every day ... just simple tasks or assignments. The question is, how do we address these tasks? Look at the double helix and see where you are. Are you passive? If you are, you will discover you become indifferent, then bored and withdrawn, and finally you will feel dissatisfied. However, if you address each task, each assignment, with action you will find that you become interested, you are able to concentrate and become totally involved."

Not everyone reading this book will become an expert in hair extension services, because not all of you will want to have this particular specialty. Again, like a doctor, you can practice general medicine or you can specialize. However, even if you practice general cosmetology, you need to *understand* the *specializations* available in your field.

When you start this book, I *know* there are some tasks you may not like to do. There will be some things that you will want to skip over. I hope you will view each chapter, each subject – looking for ways, becoming aware of all the ways that you can improve, even in the skills you already have. I hope you will take action and go up the double helix.

"It's a game that you can play with yourself with you as your only opponent. Prove to yourself that you are capable of accomplishing so much more, that you can do so much better than you are doing," encourages Dr. Ryl. Things you do every day – you can do even better!

For most of my adult life, a great portion of my income has come from the beauty industry. The material in this book is not truly original, for as you will see, there really is not much new under the sun – only new and better ways of doing things.

I am proud to be able to share with you the culmination of knowledge and experiences of many successful professionals in our industry. I know you'll enjoy entering into another dimension – *The Fourth Dimension*.

Charlotte Jayne

Charlotte Jayne

ACKNOWLEDGMENTS

I am the storyteller – sharing with you the ideas and the work of many people. There are so many to thank, I'm afraid there is no way I can list everyone.

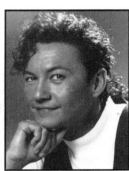
Lee Anthony
Creative Director

However, there are some people who deserve special mention. First I'd like to thank the stylists who were actively involved in the research, testing and production of this book. Without the many, many hours of work by Lee Anthony this book would not have been as complete. He was the Creative Director, designing the styles for all the case studies. Then, for each chapter, he personally followed the instructions, word for word, and led workshops of stylists and non-stylists, testing each technique for accuracy. In addition, he tested the instructions to see if they could be understood as written. Thank you, Lee, for your dedication and assistance!

In alphabetical order, the stylists who did the styles for the pictures in this book are:

Lee Anthony

James Cristopher Chan

Douglas Kovalcik

Keiko Shino

The stylists who worked as assistants for this shoot are:

Carol Ray
Donna Ramski
Beka Ledford
Kurt Lederman

There are a number of stylists who did special assignments, shared their techniques and business approaches, provided pictures and some even did video tapes. These stylists are (in alphabetical order):

Tammie Bowser

Diana Calderon

Jeannie Glover

Margaret Hawkins

Carrie Leger

Jeffrey Paul

Zina Paul

Eugenie Uboh

Kathleen Zielinski

Some more of the special people: Eileen Bernard for sharing her many years of experience in the beauty industry; Mary Sue Musser for teaching me color and about how teachers teach; Bonnie Overstreet for her support and knowledge; John Gaito for sharing his knowledge and for his fun approach to the business; Dorothy McKinley Soressi for always being there to answer questions; Keiko Shino for the years of sharing; Carol Kimble Jacob for her most informative and helpful review; Lisa Densmore and Lucy Diaz for being such willing "testers"; Catherine Frangie, the "gentle" editor whose ideas and support started this whole thing and saw it through to the last page.

I'd like to give special thanks to Mr. CK Chao, owner of CK Hair International. Thank you for nearly 20 years of working together in this industry. I'd also like to thank his employees for allowing me to photograph them.

Thanks to Marcie Gonzalez for her assistance on the illustrations. This book would have never been done without the personal support and assistance of Leann Dake for the *many hours* of proofing; Jack Waller for *all* his assistance; and last but not least, for his help and support – my best friend, Roy Westlake – thank you!

Chapter 1

INTRODUCTION

WHAT IS YOUR BUSINESS?

Keeping Up Is Hard To Do

Keeping up with fashion trends is fun. It's exciting. And it's your business. Since the beginning of time, hairstyles have been one of the most important aspects of a total fashion look.

As a hairstylist, you have to be aware of every fashion whim and every emerging trend if you are to capture the mood of the day. You must be familiar with every innovation and every new procedure so you can give your clients the total fashion look they want. The Fourth Dimension is part of our business now. Keeping up – is what you are doing by reading and working with this book.

You Influence People's Lives

You, the professional stylist (or future stylist), are in the business of caring for your client's hair. Actually, it is more than that. What you do for your clients can affect their careers, even their lives.

We all know that when people recovering from an illness begin to pay attention to their personal appearance – recovery has begun. When we feel better we want to look better.

This also works in reverse. When you don't feel well, by looking better you can feel better. In 1988 a researcher at the University College in Swansea, Wales, proved medically what fashionable people have been saying for centuries – that they feel better with a new hairstyle.

Dr. Tony Lysons, a psychologist, attached electrodes to women as they were having their hair done. He proved that in addition to improved morale, his subjects' heartbeat slowed and their blood pressure went down by 5%.

Your profession is often not given the full value it deserves. Stylists themselves do not realize how much they influence the lives of their clients. When you enter into The Fourth Dimension the importance of the work you do will come into focus. Think about it – about the responsibility!

WHAT IS THE FOURTH DIMENSION?

Once There Were Three

Once there were three, three dimensions with which to work. These three dimensions are cutting, curling and coloring.

But now there is a fourth dimension, adding hair. You really can fool Mother Nature! Adding hair is part of your business too.

Hair additions serve four purposes or combinations of these purposes. These are:

1. To add length
2. To add volume
3. To create special styles
4. To replace hair that is missing

Hair additions are divided into three categories. These are:

1. Hair extensions
2. Add-ons
3. Hair replacements

Defining Hair Extensions

A hair extension service is the addition of hair or fiber to your client's existing hair. This service involves attachment techniques that allow your client to "live with" the added hair. This means that it is part of their own hair until it is time to un-do, cleanse, service and re-attach.

The materials you add to your client's hair usually consist of either human hair, synthetic fiber or a combination of both. These usually take the form of a weft or a cluster of strands of hair or fiber.

Defining Add-ons

Add-ons are usually hair items that are designed so that they can be added and removed by the client. Some of the items are called falls, wiglets, postiches, banana clips and so on. They can be made of human hair, synthetic fiber or a combination of both.

Defining Hair Replacements

Hair replacements are "units" that are attached to your client's hair or head. These units will either replace or augment missing hair or may cover up your client's own hair.

Hair replacements may be made from human hair, synthetic fiber or a combination of both. They take the form of a hairpiece or a full wig.

WHAT THIS BOOK IS ABOUT

This book – Hair Additions, The Fourth Dimension, covers many areas that are important to all three forms of hair additions – hair extensions, add-ons and hair replacements. Information about human hair and synthetic fibers, perming and coloring apply to all hair additions. Chapter 10, Sales and Marketing, is appropriate for all these services.

However, since add-ons and hair replacements have been around for a longer period of time, this book is written primarily about the newest aspect of hair additions – hair extension services.

WHO WANTS/NEEDS HAIR ADDITION SERVICES?

Fashion – Achieving the Look

The most obvious reason for adding hair is for fashion, for achieving the look. Of course, this could mean just having hair for someone who has none, or adding length for people who either can't wait to grow their hair long or who simply can't grow long hair.

For the fun-fashion look, there is nothing like adding some hair or fiber! Fuller, thicker hair – that lovely healthy-hair look that so few men and women really have – is now available to almost anyone.

For that young man who is an accountant by day and a "rock star" on weekends, long hair added to his own locks can help him create the necessary image for his music career, yet save his day job.

Necessity – A Real Need

For people with medical problems, adding hair can mean a great deal. Individuals going through chemotherapy and people with chronic illnesses have special needs. Their lives have been changed in a negative way through no fault of their own. Trying to live "normal" lives, or even greater than that, trying to face their own extraordinary personal challenges, requires drawing on strengths from within and from without.

You can help them with the positive external influences in their lives. In these cases, beginning with hair extensions is the best way to work into the business of hair replacements.

The Bread-And-Butter Business

There is a group of clients who may very well end up being the bread-and-butter part of the hair extension service business. These are men and women over forty years of age who need to add volume to their hair. Using 100% human hair extensions that hold their curl and perfectly match your clients' hair can help your clients reduce their at home care needs. (A style that stays!) And, above all, your client will look younger.

The second group of bread-and-butter clients is those who never used to be clients at all. Women and men with baby-fine, thin hair now can have natural-looking lovely hair. Once they have hair extensions they'll never live without them! Hair – gorgeous, lovely hair!

We Want What We Don't Have

Probably the reason hair additions, either extensions or replacements, are part of our business now and are here to stay, is that it is human nature to want what we don't have. If we are tall, we wish we were shorter. If we are short, we wish we were taller. If we have straight hair, we wish we had curly hair. If we have curly hair, we wish we could have straight hair. And so on...

HAIR HAS NO SEX – HAIR HAS NO RACE

Oh No, We're Special

"Oh, you've got to be kidding. My hair is not like other people's!" "Boys don't have hair like girls." "White people don't have hair like black people." And, on and on.

The truth is, yes we are all special. We are all different. Professionals should know that their business consists of treating each person, each case as an individual!

What Is The Same

All hair is made up of three separate layers. These are the medulla, the cortex and the cuticle.

Medulla
The medulla, made up of soft keratin, is in the middle of the hair shaft and usually consists of a column of cells two, three or four rows wide. However, some hair may even be missing the medulla. The medulla may be missing as a result of genetics, a person's health or medications. The medulla's function is unknown.

Cortex
The next layer on a hair is the cortex. This comprises 75% to 90% of the shaft and is the most important layer. It is the cortex that determines the strength, direction of growth, size and texture of the hair. This is the layer that contains the color and the curl of the hair. As a result, this is the layer that is affected when changing the color or curl of hair.

Cuticle
Last is the outside layer, the cuticle. This layer protects the cortex, it is the "outer skin" of hair. The cuticle usually has five, six or seven layers of scales. Some hair, such as Chinese hair, most commonly used for the wefts for hair extensions, may have as many as eleven layers.

INTRODUCTION

What Is Different

What is different includes things you can see and things you can't.

Growth patterns are different.
Growth speeds are different.
Hair regrowth is different.
Colors are different.
Curl patterns are different.
The "inner" health of the hair is different.
The care for the hair is also different.

Why Such a Strong Statement?

Think about it. As a professional stylists, what do you do to deal some of the differences?

Hair that is *straight* has both the hydrogen and sulphur bonds in a straight position. When straight hair is curled with chemicals, first the bonds in the cortex are broken with a permanent waving solution. Then, after neutralizing and unwinding, most H and S bonds have reformed and stretched into a waved position.

Hair that is *curly* has both H and S bonds holding polypeptide chains in position. When changing curly hair with chemicals, first all the H bonds and most of the S bonds are broken. This chemical reaction begins to relax the curl. Then, after neutralizing, most of the H and S bonds have been reformed and are realigned into a straight position.

Hair that is *dark* can be lightened. Hair that is *light* can be darkened.

Hair that is *long* can be made shorter. And now, hair that is *short* or *thin* can be made longer or fuller.

When it comes to being a professional, if you *know hair*, if you know your busines, *hair has no sex* and *hair has no race*.

Time To Change!

Our industry, on the whole, is really just beginning to understand this. For the past ten years stylists have been servicing both female and male clientele. Finally, we are beginning to service all types of hair. A client's hair properties can be evaluated exactly as that – hair properties. They are a result of:

heredity
internal influences (diet, medications, hormones)
external influences (chemical services, environment, etc)

Once you have accepted the premise that hair has no sex and hair has no race, you can expand your skills to utilize your knowledge of how to work with all types of hair.

WHY NOW?

It's New – Yet It's Not

Actually, hair extensions are a new service only in a manner of speaking. The use of hair additions and adornments goes back as far as recorded history. And to understand the reason behind today's fashion trends, we should start by examining the history of hair fashions.

The early Egyptians apparently refined the idea of braiding hair and attaching decorations to these braids. Often class was identified by the type of hairstyle and type of attachments (extensions) to the hairstyle. Workers in the field might be without clothes, but their hairstyle identified their tribe, their class or their rank.

The Egyptians also wore wigs as a form of protection from the elements. Later in France, during Marie Antoinette's days, elaborate wigs were a necessary fashion item for the ruling class. Throughout history, hair additions have been in and out of fashion.

In the late 1950s and early '60s, wigs, falls and wiglets were really a big item. But by the mid-60s, the wig boom was over and had trickled down to practically nothing. Where there had been five hundred wig manufacturers, soon there were fewer than twenty.

What Is Different?

Hair additions, in the form of hair extensions, add-ons and hair replacements, are here to stay. There are a lot of reasons why these services will become part of our industry now and not fade away as they did in the 1960s. Some of these reasons are:

Better Products
There have been advances in the processing of human hair, in the manufacturing of synthetic fibers and of hair additions.

Improved Distribution
In the '60s, several factors influenced the distribution of hairgoods. The product skipped the professional market, and the direct-to-consumer market was quickly glutted with more product than could possibly be used. Now, there are fewer people in the chain of distribution. And, above all – there is a concentrated effort to keep the business more on a professional level – avoiding the "hair hat" end of the business. In addition, in the United States, we have made tremendous advancements since the '60s in communications and transportation.

Better Communications
Now, you the stylist, can call a toll-free number from anywhere in the USA and Canada and have merchandise delivered to you the next day. This advancement directly relates to the success of today's hair addition business. Keeping a complete inventory at many locations and having money tied up in that inventory have been virtually eliminated. Being

INTRODUCTION

able to provide prompt, customized services for your clients is now possible because of advanced communications and transportation capabilities that did not exist twenty years ago.

Education
This is the major reason why hair additions are here to stay. When the wig boom was here in the '60s, there was little or no related education. The entire business bypassed a majority of the professional end of our business. It was not entirely the fault of hairstylists. Manufacturers were either not forthright about what their product or not knowledgeable enough about hairstyling to relay any valuable information to our industry. Right from the beginning, the business in the '60s was geared to the retail market. There was a product but no relationship to the ongoing needs of service and hair care needs. What happened in the '60s has served to show us the way for the future.

New Techniques
This could be considered as part of the above category – Education. But, it's more than just advanced education. It's about people in our industry reaching out – surpassing themselves in developing new and better ways to do things. More than ever, stylists have shown their inventiveness and their increased understanding of products, tools and clients' needs.

WHY AND HOW IT AFFECTS THE INDUSTRY

Why This Book

The major objective of this book is to help inform all people involved in our industry about today's uses of hair additions, specifically, hair extension services, truly the fourth dimension of our business. And, to help licensed stylists who are willing to invest the time and learn how to do hair extension services.

Expansion into hair addition services will have far-reaching effects on all aspects of our industry. Sounds rather dramatic, doesn't it?

Well, let's look at what is happening in our industry and in our society, and I think you'll agree.

Why a Change Is Needed – Issues to Consider

There are fewer professionals to service more people. We are facing a crisis in our industry. There simply will not be enough stylists to serve all the people needing their services. There are fewer and fewer people available to train. The reasons for this are:

- The baby boom is over, so there are literally fewer people available to go into our profession.

- There are more options for people who would ordinarily join our industry. Now, people who are artistic and self-motivated can go into the broad area of computers and other service-oriented fields.

Income for licensed stylists has not kept up with inflation. It's true. There is more money available in other service-oriented fields than currently is available in our industry. For the hours worked, the risks taken and the education required, licensed stylists are making less than they would if they went into other fields.

There are exceptions. There *are* stylists who are making an excellent income! These exceptions, these stylists, are individuals who have continued to expand their skills and services – and individuals who have learned better time management and people skills. (But this could be the subject of another book.)

Now, here is a new service, hair additions, that easily increases the per-hour income of a licensed stylist. This new service requires the skilled services of a knowledgeable professional.

How Hair Additions Will Change Our Industry

Hair addition services assure more income per hour than any other salon service. They require advanced education, which may help to upgrade our industry.

More effective use of time and better people skills are required to attract clients for this service. An emphasis throughout our industry on improvement of these skills will have a positive effect.

With the excitement caused by hair addition services, both from within our industry and from the general public, continuing education will become more and more important. If more stylists devote more time to learning, to improving, to growing – this will also have an uplifting effect on our entire industry. As there are more advanced education classes, there will be greater demand for more and better courses.

DEFINITION OF TERMS

Re-Definition Is Required

Today's hair extension services are the result of a progression from previous techniques – employing specialized terms. Because of this, it is necessary to redefine some terms and create new ones as needed.

As an example, you may hear the term "hair weaving" to describe hair extension services. Actually, hair weaving describes just one way of attaching hair extensions. The best way to define terms is to use Webster's dictionary as the source.

INTRODUCTION

Important Words to Learn

Weave
"To form, as a textile, by interlacing yarns. To move to and fro, up and down, or in an intricate course."

Extension
"Act of extending, or state of being extended ... an addition."

Braid
"To weave, interlace, or entwine together, as three or more strands."

Weft
"A weft is a weaving, a thing woven."

Track
"A track is a path or course laid out."

Discussion of the Words

As you can see, the words weave, braid, and even the word weft, can easily be interchanged.

The term hair weaving is used in two different ways. The *first* use of the term *hair weaving* means to make a weft and other hair goods. The tools that are used date back more than two hundred years – the hackle, drawing cards, weaving poles. To make a hand-tied weft, loose hair is woven between three threads. The end result, the weft, looks like a hula skirt. Today most wefts are machine made, but the term weft still applies.

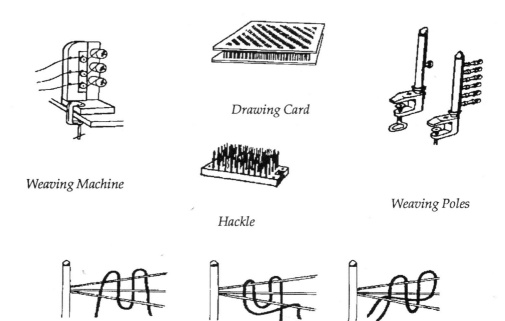

Weaving Machine

Drawing Card

Hackle

Weaving Poles

Hand-Tied wefts made by weaving hair between three threads

The *second* use of the term *hair weaving* means to make a track on the client's head. This is done using three threads from three spools that are placed on a "weaving machine" or on weaving poles. The client's hair is woven between three threads. This creates a "track" on which wefts can be attached.

The word "track" is important because that is where you place the weft. The type of method you use to create a track depends on the technique you feel is best for the situation. We'll discuss these techniques later on. When you are designing the placement pattern, you are deciding where you will track (place the tracks) on your client's head.

Today, hair weaving, making a track, tracking, braiding – all are terms that are used. The art of extending hair involves a multitude of techniques. And, taking into account the creativity and inventiveness of the professional hairstylist, I know that as time goes on, we'll see more ways being developed.

Micro Filler Fiber Braid
This is a braided track using the micro filler fiber braiding technique. The weft of hair is then sewn on to this track.

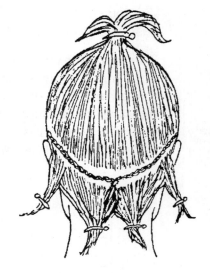

Individual Braids.
A track for the individual braiding technique is the parting where the braids are placed.

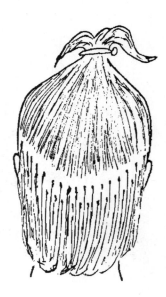

INTRODUCTION

Bonding
For the bonding technique, a track is also the parting, the place where the is bonded to the client's hair.

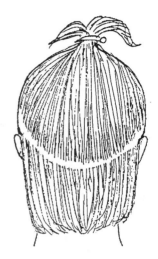

Weaving.
A track, again the place where the weft of hair will be attached (sewn), is made by capturing hair in three threads when doing the weaving technique.

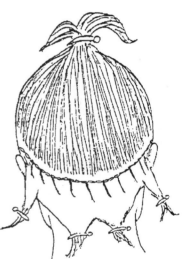

INFORMATION ABOUT HUMAN HAIR

Where Does the Hair Come From?

The first question I'm asked is, "Where does the hair come from?"

Would you believe, I've seen advertisements that say – "... from our hair farm ..." No, not hair farms. Here are the facts! There are only three major sources of human hair: China, India and Europe.

Hair from Europe is less readily available and the quality is less dependable. There is a very limited supply. As a matter of fact, there is only one small country in Europe currently collecting and selling hair. This hair is also dark in color, which means it must be decolorized (bleached) to lighter colors, it varies a great deal in quality and it is very expensive. The second largest source of human hair is from India. The hair is usually of good quality, is soft in texture and has a slight natural wave.

However, the majority of human hair comes from China. This is because China is the only country that has a formalized method of collecting hair. The Chinese have always considered all hair, including human hair, a natural resource and have collected it. They also have had an active trade in hair as a commodity.

The selling of their hair has been a source of income for people in China for hundreds of years. The Chinese people cut their hair and even save the hair that comes out on their combs. The "hair collectors" travel from village to village trading items for the hair. This hair is then taken to warehouses throughout China where it is separated and graded.

Hair Has Been Used in Many Ways

Throughout the history of China, hair has had many uses. In the early history of China, hair was used to make protective vests. This was done by taking hair, wetting it, then matting it. When the hair dried after being matted, it was made into a protective garment or shield. No one could get a sword through it. Human hair has also been used as insulation in houses. Even today, mattresses and rugs in China are made from poorer quality human hair. The original hair nets were made from strands of human hair. The original cross-hair sight on a rifle was two hairs crossed in the glass. Artist and industrial brushes have been made of human hair from China. And, of course, most of you are aware of Manikins, wefts, wigs, etc. that are made with Chinese human hair.

What Is Indonesian Hair?

You may have heard the term "Indonesian hair." There really is no such thing because there is very little hair available from Indonesia. Actually, the term was created to get around a political situation. Until 1974, there was an embargo in the United States on all merchandise from China. To get around this, hair from China was sent to other countries first and then imported into the USA as "Indonesian hair".

You Can't Believe All Labeling

It is unfortunate, but you need to understand that there are unscrupulous people in the hair-trading business. They label hair 100% Human Hair, or even 100% European Hair, when in fact, it is not. The hair may pass through many countries and many people before you purchase it so that the end seller may not be aware of the deception.

How Can You Check For 100% Human Hair?

How can you find out if the hair you purchased is 100% Human Hair? There are three tests you can perform to determine if the hair you have purchased is 100% human hair.

Burn Test
Be sure to use common sense when conducting this test. Fire is nothing to take lightly.

Human hair will maintain a flame. It will burn. At the ends, where the hair burned, you will see that it turned to ashes.

Synthetic fibers (most of those allowed in the United States) will not burn. They melt instead. When you feel the ends, where you have applied the flame, the fiber residue crumbles between your fingers.

When you do the burn experiment, you will notice a difference in the odor between the 100% human hair and the synthetic fiber. However, the burn test may not be conclusive if the wefts are blended. That is, they are part human hair and part synthetic fiber. You will have to use the other tests to make your determination.

Perm Test
Following manufacturer's instructions, wrap and perm a strand of synthetic fiber and a strand of 100% human hair.

Synthetic fiber will not take a perm, whereas human hair will have a curl formation after applying a permanent wave solution.

Color Test
The last test is to color (or bleach) the hair. Synthetic fibers will not change color with professional tints or bleaches whereas 100% human hair will.

Processing Hair for Wefts and Other Items

Hair that is collected naturally has different characteristics and is different in quality. It's just like with your clients' hair, some have strong healthy hair, others have damaged or weak hair.

Hair must first be graded, then bundled. There are generally two types of hair used in hair goods:

1. Root-Turned Hair
2. Processed Hair

Root-turned hair is also called "Cut" hair because the hair is as it was cut from the person's head. This means all the roots and ends are going in the same direction. This type of hair is now in limited supply.

Processed hair has been treated so that it will not tangle. To "process" hair, the cuticle must be stripped.

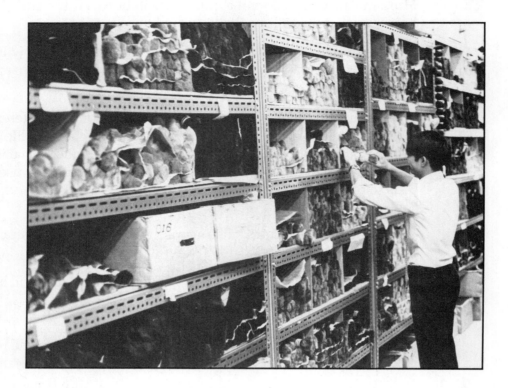

First, hair is collected and graded. Lower grades of hair are used to make mattresses, rugs and industrial brushes.

Next, hair is weighed and bundled. Then it is stored until it is ready to be processed.

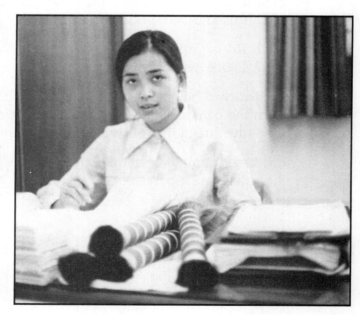

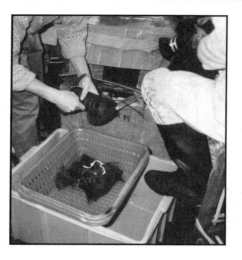

When it is time to process the hair, the strings on the bundles are cut and the hair is placed in plastic baskets.

It is then thoroughly washed. It may have been stored for many years and traveled thousands of miles. (Hair is stored so it can get moisture from the air, never in plastic.)

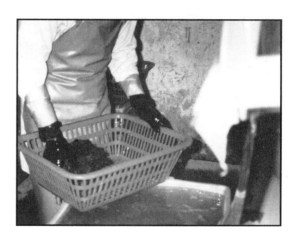

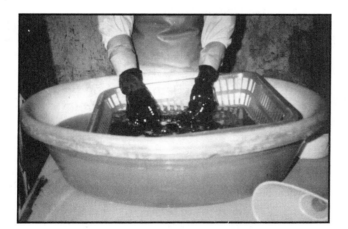

The hair is then placed in a solution of muriatic acid.

To strip the cuticle just the right amount is tricky. Too much and the hair is over-processed. Just like any over processed hair, it will be damaged. It cannot successfully accept additional chemical services and will break. If too little cuticle is removed, the hair will tangle and mat.

Stripping the cuticle is done by dipping the hair into muriatic acid to soften the cuticle. Then the hair is gathered into small bundles and, using something like a fingernail brush, it is scrubbed by hand to remove part of the cuticle.

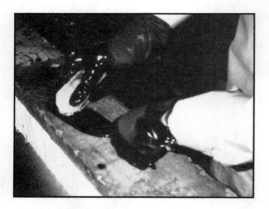

After being dipped in muriatic acid the hair is scrubbed to remove part of the cuticle.

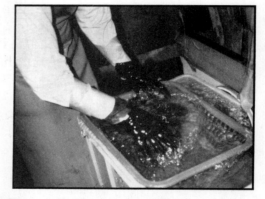

Next the hair is rinsed in a solution to neutralize the acid.

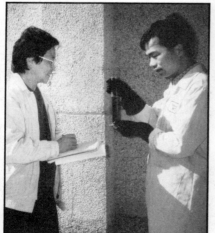

Since all Chinese and Indian hair is black, to achieve other colors the next step of processing is to decolorize (bleach) the hair. The chemists at the factory need to check the bleaching chemicals, the water and the temperature.

Much of the hair that is sold has first been lightened and then dyed with chrome dyes. Usually, dyed hair is not marked as dyed hair, whereas hair that is not dyed usually is marked as non-dyed hair.

If you are going to do chemical services to hair goods, it is important that you use non-dyed hair.

What Kind of Hair Is Best?

Another question I'm often asked is, "What kind of hair is best to use?" To answer that question, we need to look at all the factors. First, European hair is now in very limited supply and, as a result, is very expensive. Next, the softer texture of the more expensive European hair may not be appropriate – may not necessarily achieve the desired result of fuller, thicker hair.

Again, you need to be confident of your source for hair. Unfortunately, it is difficult to identify kinds of hair. Indian hair that is processed well is often sold as European hair. One clue to identifying Indian hair is that the longest Indian hair generally available is 16" and it has a natural wave.

Actually, there probably is not a "best" kind of hair to use, whether it be European, Chinese or Indian. The best kind of hair for you to use is hair that accomplishes the results you want at a price that is appropriate. Besides being assured that the hair is 100% human hair, the two most important aspects to know about the hair you purchase are:

1. Is it correctly processed so it won't mat or tangle?

2. Do you know if the hair is dyed or non-dyed?

Ways Hair Is Sold

You can purchase hair several ways. Bulk hair is loose, not sewn on a weft. When you purchase hair "in bulk" you can use it only for individual braiding or interweaving techniques. This hair is difficult to perm or color simply because it is loose.

The other way you can purchase hair is in a weft (either hand-tied or machine-made). Hair in a weft can be colored and permed and can then be cut from the weft to be used as loose hair.

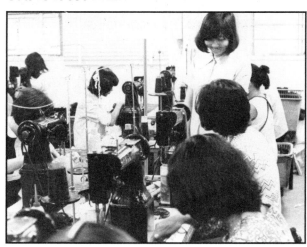

Wefts are made using specially designed sewing machines. The hair for each weft is first weighed. The amount of hair, by weight, is one aspect of a machine-made weft that is almost always consistent.

The loose hair is then sewn together. This picture shows what is considered the first stitching. The hair is then folded according to the design of the weft. Because the hair is hand-fed through the sewing machine, the width of the weft may vary from 2" to 4", and the finished length by as much as 1" to 2".

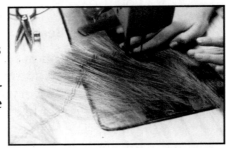

The advantage of a hand-tied weft over a machine-made weft is that it is thinner at the top. The disadvantages are that it is very delicate and will not last as long as a machine-made weft. It cannot be used for the bonding attachment technique. Machine-made wefts are thicker and are more suitable for bonding. They will not unravel when cut to match your tracking.

The workmanship on both hand-tied and machine-made wefts varies greatly. Some hand-tied wefts are made with large clumps of hair and, as a result, are not much thinner than some machine-made wefts. Wefts are sewn in many different ways, with different "fold-overs." By fold-over, I mean what is literally the seam, the place where the hair is captured. The amount of hair captured in the fold-over affects the thickness at the top of the weft. For hair used in the crown or side area of a style, this may be an important consideration. Some wefts are single-density, whereas others are double-density. Single-density means that the weft has been sewn only one time and the fold-over hair is exposed. Double-density wefts have been sewn so that the short fold-over hair is captured in the middle of the weft.

Being Informed Is Important

Knowing about and understanding the hair you use for extensions is as helpful and as important as knowing and understanding the products you use to service your clients. This may be difficult because few vendors of hair goods really know exactly where their products come from. Many of them are not stylists nor are they knowledgeable about our industry. Many of them are simply salespeople.

One stylist in Southern California paid a painfully high price for his ignorance about hair goods when he lost a $500 judgment in small-claims court. His client sued him for using Chinese hair. Another stylist convinced the client that European hair was superior to Chinese hair and cost only $50 more. The client then sued her previous stylist, stating that "European Wavy" hair was European hair (for only $50 more) whereas he had used Chinese hair. The stylist tried to explain that the term "European Wavy" is sometimes used to describe pre-permed hair, which is Chinese hair. But the judge, like the client, did not understand. I spent some time with the stylist explaining the history of hair, definitions of terms, etc. At the time of this writing, the stylist has filed an appeal and I hope that he wins, now that he has facts to present and is better prepared to educate the judge.

INFORMATION ABOUT SYNTHETIC FIBERS

Five Basic Materials Used For Synthetic Fibers

1. *Nylon*

Nylon is a very shiny fiber and is now used mainly for dolls' hair.

2. *Polypropylene*

Polypropylene is flammable and is not legal to use here in the United States. It is currently used only in underdeveloped countries for cheap carnival wigs.

3. *Polyester*

Polyester is also used for wigs, but in very small quantities.

4. and 5. *P.V.C.* and *Modacrylic*

P.V.C. and Modacrylic are the main fibers used for wigs today. These fibers are easy to "program," that is, to permanently set in a curl. Permanent curl is set by wetting the fiber, then placing in an oven at 212 degrees Fahrenheit (90 degrees Centigrade) for one hour. These fibers closely resemble human hair. P.V.C. is more suitable for long and wavy styles, whereas Modacrylic is more suitable for short and curly styles. Today most synthetic "hair" goods are a blend of P.V.C. and Modacrylic fibers in a ratio that best suits a particular style.

Making Synthetic Fibers To Resemble Human Hair

As you know, human hair has a rough cuticle and is never completely round or "perfect" in any way. Synthetic fibers, however, are "perfect" and cannot really look like human hair, since they reflect light differently.

Fibers are available in different diameters and are "cross sections" (described as C type and Y type) to help reflect light differently and reduce the shiny nature of fibers.

In addition, when making "hair" goods with synthetic fibers, some manufacturers add different coating materials to the fibers which will create different effects in the look and feel of the fibers.

Most fibers are dyed to 33 three different colors. These solid colors are then blended to create more natural-looking "human hair" colors.

Synthetic Fibers Used in Hair Extensions

Some stylists use synthetic fibers for their hair extension services. There is one type of service for which synthetic fibers is usually preferred. That is the exposed braid style.

However, synthetic fibers are generally not the best product to use for hair extensions.

Synthetic fibers cannot be colored to match your client's hair, nor can they be permed to match. The texture difference is often obvious. But probably the most important reason is that synthetic fibers do not hold up as well as 100% human hair. Friction causes synthetic fibers to mat and tangle.

Another important thing you should consider is that the cost of the hair or fiber is really the least expensive aspect of hair extension services. This service is your signature – the result of your time and skills. It's your time and your skills for which your client is paying. When considering whether to use human hair or synthetic fiber, think about the finished product. Aren't you looking for the best? Aren't you trying to give your client the best you can?

When it comes to hair extension services, there really is no substitute for 100% human hair. In all my years of experience in the business, I've worked with both synthetic fibers and human hair. For hair extensions, I can recommend only 100% human hair for a number of reasons. But the main reason is that when you are adding to a client's own hair, to add anything other than 100% human hair is like mixing oil and water.

ATTACHMENT TECHNIQUES

If hair extension services were easy to do, everybody would be doing them. As it is, there are a lot of stylists trying, and they should be given special recognition. But in all truth, it takes more than just trying – it takes true dedication and continuing practice. Hair extensions are a real specialty. Not every stylist can do hair extensions. It is estimated that only about 3% of currently licensed stylists will be able to provide hair extension services successfully.

Why do I say that? Because not every stylist will take the time to learn and practice all the skills that are required. In addition, hair extension services require a different kind of commitment – you will work your book entirely differently.

INTRODUCTION

Mary Sue Musser taught me a very important word you too should remember. The word is HAIR. We really are in the HAIR business. And the word means:

How
Am
I
Responsible

How Am I Responsible? If at all times we ask ourselves this question, we can avoid using techniques that may not be advisable for a particular client's hair. Remembering your responsibility toward your client and your own reputation, can save you a lot of grief in the long run.

There are many attachment methods. Since the subject is so involved, I decided to discuss in detail only three of them. These three techniques are ones that I consider basic, are safe and are the most commonly used.

Bonding

The easiest attachment technique is called bonding. The product used to attach the wefts to the client's own hair should be a natural product made from latex (rubber from rubber trees).

Although it is the easiest method, it is also the least dependable. Bond loses its adhesive properties when mixed with oil. As a result, clients with oily scalps or those who use hair preparations that are oily cannot have wefts bonded to their own hair.

Bond is applied to the weft and to the client's own hair. The attachment technique is similar to applying strip eyelashes. (See Chapter 3.)

Braid Tracking and Sewing

Probably the most basic attachment technique is the braided track with the weft sewn onto the track. If a client's hair is long enough to braid, this technique is probably the best and most durable to use.

A braided track. The weft is sewn onto this track. Tracks are placed to create the desired style. (See Chapter 5.)

Individual Braids

The individual braid technique is also important to learn. It is more time-consuming and may be done all over the head or in selected areas. It's an excellent technique for people with thinning hair. It's a very good technique to use for a fashion-statement hairstyle. As an example, if you want to add a second color to a client's hair without doing any chemical services, you can do this by doing individual braids. In one of the styles shown in this book, Larry wanted some long hair in the front. This too is an excellent application for the individual braids. (See Chapter 6.)

Weaving Thread Tracks

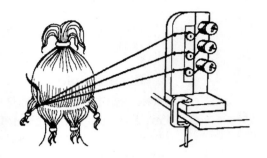

This technique is the origin of the term hair weaving. It is considered an advanced technique. A track is made by weaving the client's own hair through three threads. Or when two threads are used, it often is called "cabling."

Wefts, add-ons or hair replacements are sewn to these tracks. The weaving machine is simply a device that holds three spools of thread. It sounds like some kind of machine that will do the weaving for you, doesn't it? Too bad, it doesn't do anything but hold the thread and help apply tension to the thread. The machine needs to be placed above and to the right of your client's head. A track is woven using your client's own hair and three threads.

This is a more difficult technique to learn, is difficult to do on straight hair and most salons do not have the space required to properly place the weaving machine.

The weaving technique (and cabling, which is the same technique but with only two threads) may play a more important role in some forms of hair replacement attachment. I've not included weaving/cabling techniques in this book. However, once you are into the business of adding hair – chances are you'll be expanding your skills and your services to include hair replacements. So you will want to learn this technique.

Other Techniques

There are a number of other techniques used in hair extension services. One of these is called interlock weaving. It is a technique where loose hair (rather than a weft) is woven into the track. The track can be made either by making a micro-braid or by weaving a track with threads. I consider interlock weaving an advanced technique and one that is more applicable for extremely curly hair but difficult on straight hair. As a result, I've not included it in this book.

Other techniques involve crossing over two, three or four strands of hair or fiber interwoven within the client's own hair. Then the hair or fiber is braided or twisted together and is often affixed by using a glue or wax. I have not included these techniques in the book. Most of them are too time-consuming when compared to the other techniques you will learn here. But, more important, many of these techniques are hazardous to the client's own hair, particularly if not done correctly. By the word hazardous, I mean that either the technique used for attachment can damage the client's own hair and/or the finished style is too difficult for the client to maintain. <u>If the hairstyle is not manageable by the client and if the technique used does not allow the client to properly cleanse her or his scalp or hair, then the service should not be done.</u>

One of the more popular techniques that I also have not included in this book involves affixing clusters of "loose" hairs (or fibers) to clusters of the client's hair by melting a wax/glue at the point where the added hair/fiber and the client's hair meet. Although this technique is faster than making individual braids, there are too many hazards involved. In addition to over-doing the application of the wax/glue, there is an ever greater risk of <u>client mismanagement</u>. I've seen clients with large matted messes the size of a baseball in the backs of their heads which resulted in bald spots the size of a quarter or fifty-cent piece. There are a number of reasons this problem occurs, but since there are so many other options, so many other techniques to use, I'm excluding this one from the book.

Which Technique Is Best?

The answer to the question, "Which technique is best?" is – the technique that meets the following requirements:

Appropriateness
A technique or combination of techniques should provide the type of style that is appropriate for your client. This means: Is the technique correct for your client's type of hair, your client's own hair length and the length of hair being attached? Your client's lifestyle? Your client's finished style requirements?

Manageability
Techniques should allow your clients the maximum "control" of their own home hair-care activities.

Affordability
Do you, as a stylist, have the time to first, become an expert in this technique, and second, have the ability to manage your book for the time required for application and ongoing client in-salon maintenance? Also, is the technique affordable for the client? Do your clients have the time required for the services and for the home care? Will the clients get their money's worth? <u>Will you be paid appropriately for the cost of your supplies, your skills and your time?</u>

SUMMARY

Until recently, stylists have worked in three dimensions – cutting, curling and coloring. Now there is The Fourth Dimension – adding hair for volume and/or length. It is a service for which there is a great need and a growing demand. Stylists who apply themselves to learning it can be assured of a more lucrative and satisfying career.

Since synthetic fibers simply do not work as well, 100% human hair is highly recommended for hair extensions. Human hair comes from China, India and Europe. It is sometimes mixed with synthetic fibers and mislabeled 100% human hair, but there are some ways to ascertain whether or not it is. It is important for the stylist to know their source and feel confident about the product.

Several attachment techniques will be described in later chapters. It is essential that the stylist know all of them, even if only one or two are used. With a background of information and practice the stylist will be able to sell a client on hair extensions, always keeping this motto in mind:

How
Am
I
Responsible

Chapter 2

BRAIDING AND SEWING TRACKS

INTRODUCTION

You Must Learn the Scales to Play

Right here, in this chapter, begin the basics for hair extension services. It's like learning to play an instrument. You must first learn to play the scales and then practice and practice. For hair extension services, you must learn to make specific kinds of braids and then practice and practice making them.

It may sound dumb – but I guarantee you – if you don't already know how to make micro-braids, and particularly micro filler fiber braids, with just the right amount of tension – you may find this task frustrating.

To be honest with you, trying to learn how to correctly braid a track from a book is even more of a challenge. Give it your best shot. However, if you can't master the technique by reading this book – look for a video or a hands-on class to help you.

Four Types of Practice Braids

Before you can even begin making tracks you'll need to learn what I call practice braids. The four types of practice braids you will learn are:

1. Under braid

2. Under filler fiber braid

3. Under braid on scalp

4. Under filler fiber braid on scalp (micro filler fiber braid)

In this chapter you will learn how to do these braids. I can't emphasize enough that this is the foundation for two very important techniques used in attaching hair extensions. You need to be able to do these braids for both the Braid and Sew attachment technique and for the Individual Braiding technique.

ADVANTAGES AND DISADVANTAGES

Advantages

There are several advantages to the Braid and Sew attachment technique. Probably the first and most important advantage is that, if done correctly, it is the safest of all the attachment techniques. In addition, it does not require special equipment and the supplies that are required are easy to obtain. When you are an expert, well practiced in making micro-braids, you will discover that they can be done quite quickly.

I have known stylists (particularly male stylists who have had limited exposure to any type of braiding) who have become proficient enough to braid a track in 5 to 8 minutes. Of course, I do mean a clean, correctly executed micro-braid using a filler fiber. When these stylists began, it took them 30 minutes to do a track.

The Braid and Sew attachment technique is safe, requires no equipment, only a few supplies and is not very time consuming.

Disadvantages

The disadvantages of this technique are only a few. First, to make a track correctly takes time to learn! Yes, a lot of people can braid. A lot of people can braid fast. But, a lot of the work I've seen is not neat and clean. If a braid is done incorrectly, not clean and with incorrect tension, the problems caused can include: the client's hair may be damaged, the client may experience severe discomfort and spot baldness may occur.

Other disadvantages are related to the appropriateness of this technique relative to the client's own hair and life style. As an example, some individuals who are unable, or find it difficult, to care for their own hair could have problems. Some of the problems include: not getting the scalp clean around and in between the tracking, which may cause irritation; allowing soap or other things to be trapped in the tracking, thus causing irritation to the scalp, not getting the track (and the hair) dry after shampooing, which can cause scalp irritation and/or can mat the hair, excessive perspiration, again causing irritation, etc.

Another disadvantage of the tracking technique is that sometimes the client's hair is just too short to braid.

SUPPLIES

Introduction

If you are going to learn hair extension services, it is really important to have the necessary and appropriate supplies. Please don't try to follow the instructions in this chapter, in this book, without first getting everything together. Stop right now and get the supplies you need. Without them you'll be unnecessarily handicapping yourself.

The list of supplies you will need are:

Manikin	Small rubber bands
Manikin holder	Filler fiber
Large comb	Needles
Rattail comb	Nail file
Clips	Thread
Spray bottle of water	Speed-bond
Hair spray	Shears (a "working" pair)
A weft	

Important Warning

Do not try to learn braiding on a person's head. You will need to practice and practice and practice. You will need a Manikin to use for the hours of practice required to become proficient in hair extension services.

Also, you will need to use a Manikin and holder for many aspects of hair extension services. As an example, if you are going to custom perm the wefts for your client's hairstyle you will need the Manikin head on which to attach the weft. To assist in better communication with prospective clients, your Manikin can be very helpful for demonstration of various attachment techniques and for sales purposes.

Manikin Head and Holder

Your Manikin should have hair that is about 8" long, which is long enough yet not too long for learning how to braid tracks.

Also, you may want to purchase the new type of vacuum holder for your Manikin. This kind of holder allows you to put your Manikin on any smooth surface — which means you will be able to use the Manikin anywhere you have a smooth surface in your salon or at home. This holder is available from several sources. Ask your local beauty supply distributor.

So, before you begin anything be sure to get a Manikin and holder — they are a must!

Other Items

The large comb and rattail comb are needed to properly comb the hair and/or make your all-important partings. The clips are necessary to keep the hair you are not braiding from being caught in your work. The spray bottle of water and the hair spray are helpful in controlling the hair and/or the filler fiber.

The small rubber bands are needed to finish your braid. These you can purchase at any stationery store or your hair goods supplier. You want the smallest size available. At shops that carry supplies for horses, you can purchase different colored rubber bands. (These are used for braiding manes and tails for show horses. As a quick aside, did you know that hair extensions are often done on horses' manes and tails?)

Filler fiber is a very curly synthetic fiber. You'll recognize this as a fiber sometimes used in certain types of "ponytails". You can purchase filler fiber from most companies that sell hair goods.

The recommended needles can be purchased at your local fabric store or from your hair goods source. There is usually available a 7-needle set designed for sewing everything from sacks to sails. In this set, two are the best to use. These are the ones used for yarn crafts or for sacks and string sewing. Some stylists like to use a curved needle, but I don't recommend this because a curved needle is more difficult to control, which means the stitching may not be as neat as it could/should be.

There is only one kind of thread to use. It is a cotton covered polyester thread. It is also available at fabric stores or your supplier of hair goods. The reason this thread is preferable is because: all cotton thread will shrink and/or stretch when wet and is often not strong enough, whereas all polyester thread, fishing line, wire, etc. is too sharp and will cut the client's hair. The solution is a blend of both — cotton on the outside of the thread and polyester on the inside.

Shears, what I call a "working" pair, are needed to cut both the thread and the weft. You don't want to use your good haircutting shears. I'd suggest using about a 5" size shear. It needs to be small enough to have good control.

Speed-bond is a specific adhesive that is used in hair extension services as a means of locking individual braids. It is available from some hair goods companies and is similar to products sold in auto supply stores. (See Chapter 3.)

A weft — well, that's natural. This is the hair you'll sew onto the track.

Remember, these items should be available from your hair source.

EXERCISES

Introduction

"Exercises?" you say. Don't raise your eyebrows — they really will help. First, so many of us are really tense in the shoulders, neck and lower back areas. Before you even begin the braiding practices, it can help you to loosen up. And, after you are at it for a while — just stop and do a few of these exercises.

These particular exercises are called *The Range of Motion Exercises*. The following are reprinted with permission from PEP•USA (Parkinson's Educational Program).

A. Cervical Movements

Do the following activities sitting in a straight back chair. *Maintain good posture.* Do each movement *5 times*, counting slowly and *out loud*.

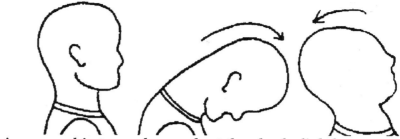

1. Bring your chin toward your chest then back slightly so you are looking toward the ceiling.

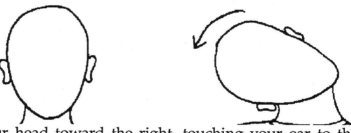

2. Bend your head toward the right, touching your ear to the right shoulder. Then repeat, touching your left ear to your left shoulder. Make sure you keep your head facing forward.

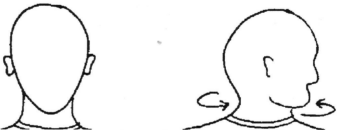

3. Turn your head to look as far to the right as possible, then to the left.

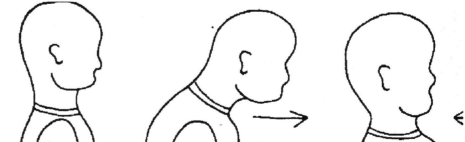

4. Push your head forward as far as possible. Then move it backward, attempting to make a double chin. Hold for 5 seconds; relax with your head in this position or near to it.

B. Shoulder Movements

Do the following activities sitting in a straight back chair. *Maintain good posture.* Do each movement *5 times*, counting slowly and *out loud*.

1. Bring your shoulders up and back (shrugging). Then relax to normal position.

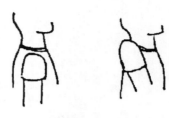

2. With arms relaxed at your side, bring your shoulders slowly into a complete circle, first up and forward, then up and back.

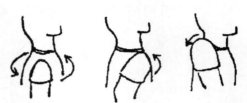

3. Keeping your arms straight, raise them overhead as far as possible, hold for a 2 counts, then relax.

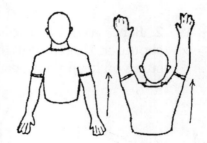

4. Keeping your arms straight, raise them out to the side and overhead, then out to the side again and back down.

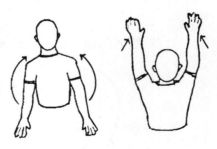

5. Place your hands behind your head and push your elbows back as far as possible (taking care not to pull your head forward). Hold this position for 2 seconds, then relax.

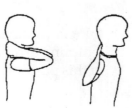

C. Elbow, Forearm, Wrist and Hand Movements

Again, do the following activities sitting in a straight back chair, *maintaining good posture*. Perform each movement *5 times*. Counting out loud and slowly helps exercise your muscles related to your voice.

1. Bend your elbows until your hands hit your shoulders. Next, straighten your arms in front of you and relax.

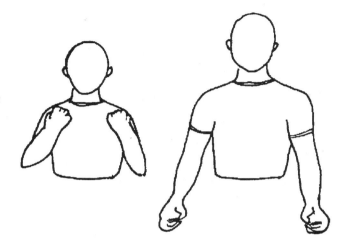

2. Holding your arms at your side and your elbows at right angles, alternately turn your palms up and down as far as possible.

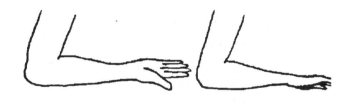

3. Keeping the same position, alternately bend your wrist up and down as far as possible.

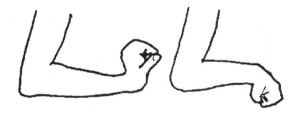

4. Next, alternately make a fist and relax your hands as far as possible.

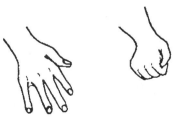

D. Hip, Knee, Ankle and Toe Movements

Still sitting in a straight back chair, do the following activities. Perform each movement *5 times*, counting slowly and *out loud*.

1. Straighten your right knee and move your foot in 3 large circles, lower your leg and repeat with the left leg.

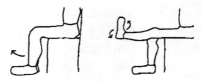

2. Keeping your left knee bent, swing your foot to the middle then out to the side. Repeat 5 times. Do the same with your right leg. Repeat 5 times.

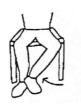 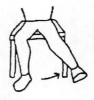

3. Holding your left foot out, point your foot down while curling your toes then bring your foot back up toward you while straightening your toes. After 5 times, switch and do the same movement with your right foot.

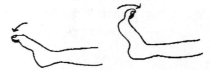

4. With your hands on your hips, slowly turn your shoulders toward the left as far as possible then toward the right. Repeat 5 times.

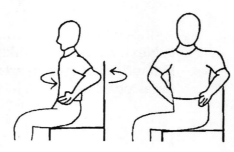

E. Trunk Movements

Perform the following exercises in a standing position. Do each movement *5 times*, counting slowly and *out loud*.

1. Place your hands on your hips. Lean forward slightly then slowly return upright. Next lean backward. At the end of 5 repetitions, concentrate on keeping good, upright posture.

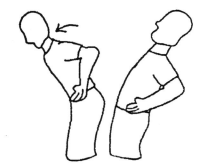

2. With your hands on your hips, lean over to the right as far as possible, then return upright. Next lean to the left as far as possible and return upright. Repeat 5 times.

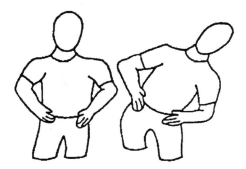

F. Leg Movements

Perform the following exercises in a standing position. You may want to use a counter or some other firm support as a handhold. Do each movement *5 times*, counting slowly and *out loud*.

1. Standing straight, alternately lift your leg as far out to the side as possible then your right leg.

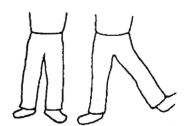

2. Standing straight, alternately straighten each leg out behind you, keeping your knee straight.

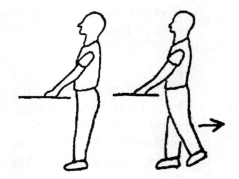

3. Slowly lower your body until your knees are bent at a right angle. Next, slowly rise all the way up onto your "tippy-toes." Repeat 5 times.

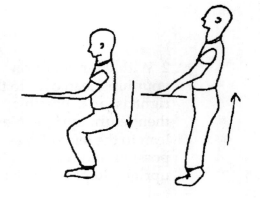

4. March, lifting your knees as high as possible. If your balance is good, let go of the support and move your arms with your legs. March!

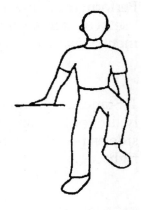

MANIKIN SET UP

It is important to learn to be comfortable. If you practice braiding correctly, one of the things you will notice is cramping in your fingers, the palms of your hands and sometimes even up your wrists, arms and shoulders. Not an exciting prospect. To get started the right way is not easy. The reason for the cramping and soreness is because you are going to be using muscles that you don't ordinarily use.

Please pay close attention to the instructions on to how to hold your fingers, hands, wrists and so on. The techniques explained were developed after years of experimentation, testing and teaching.

Set up your Manikin facing away from you. Playing some music can help because one of the tricks in learning how to braid is to set a pace – rhythm.

UNDER BRAID

Introduction

This is called an under braid because you will always be moving one strand, of the three strands, under the middle strand.

Even if you know how to braid, please follow these instructions. You will find that the first three braids you will learn in this chapter will lead you into learning how to make the perfect micro filler fiber braid.

The micro filler fiber braid is how you make tracks for the Braid and Sew technique.

Make yourself comfortable – comfortable clothes and shoes. Listen to music. Now you are ready to begin.

Hands, Fingers and Wrists

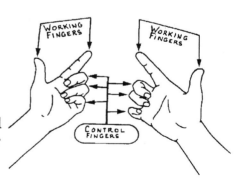

Working Fingers
These fingers are called your working fingers. They will manipulate the hair to be moved.

Control Fingers
These fingers are called your control fingers because they control the hair – holding it in place and maintaining tension as you are braiding.

Wrist Movement
Keep your wrists loose and flexible. Your wrist movements are important in helping to maintain tension, in correct positioning of the strands of hair and in the total appearance of the braid.

Make a Square

For your first practice under braid, take a 2" square section of hair at the center front of the hairline on your Manikin. Then, with clips, secure the hair that is not going to be braided.

Separate Hair

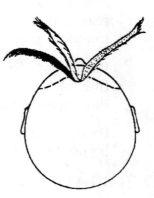

Next, divide the hair to be braided into three equal parts.

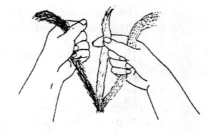

In your right hand – your right control fingers – hold the right strand.

In your right hand – your right working fingers – hold the middle strand.

In your left hand – your left control fingers – hold the left strand.

Remember to keep your wrists loose and flexible because your wrist movements are important in helping to maintain tension, in correct positioning of the strands of hair and in the total appearance of the braid.

First Cross Under

Pick Up Strand
With your left working fingers, reach under your right hand and pick up the right strand.

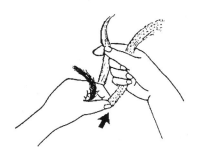

Twist Wrist
Twist your left wrist – causing your palm to face upward. This motion will pull the right strand under the center strand.

The new middle strand will now be in your left working fingers.

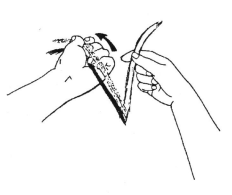

Transfer Strand
Transfer the strand in your right working fingers to your right control fingers. Maintain the tension.

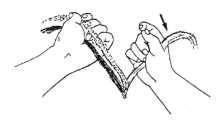

Second Cross Under

Pick Up Strand
With your right working fingers, reach under your left hand and pick up the left strand.

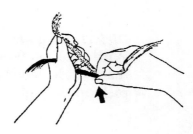

Twist Wrist
Twist your right wrist – causing your palm to face upward. This motion will pull the left strand under the center strand.

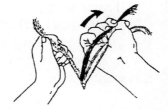

The new middle strand will now be in your right working fingers.

Transfer Strand
Transfer the strand in your left working fingers to your left control fingers. Maintain the tension.

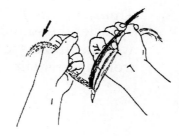

Third Cross Under

Pick Up Strand
With your left working fingers, reach under your right hand and pick up the right strand.

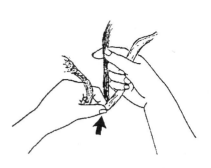

Twist Wrist
Twist your left wrist — causing your palm to face upward. This motion will pull the right strand under the center strand.

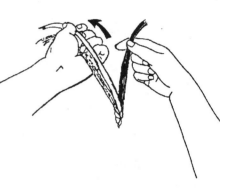

The new middle strand will now be in your left working fingers.

Transfer Strand
Transfer the strand in your right working fingers to your right control fingers. Maintain the tension.

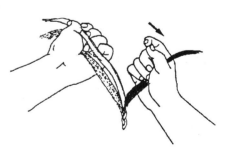

Fourth Cross Under

Pick Up Strand
With your right working fingers, reach under your left hand and pick up the left strand.

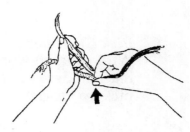

Twist Wrist
Twist your right wrist – causing your palm to face upward. This motion will pull the left strand under the center strand.

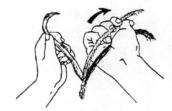

The new middle strand will now be in your right working fingers.

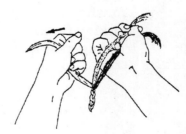

Transfer Strand
Transfer the strand in your left working fingers to your left control fingers. Maintain the tension.

Continue Braiding

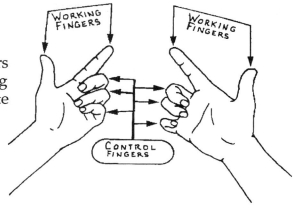

Working Fingers: These fingers are called your working fingers. They will manipulate the hair to be moved.

Control Fingers: These fingers are called your control fingers because they control the hair – holding it in place and maintaining tension as you are braiding.

Remember to use your *working fingers* to pick up the hair to be moved (braided) and your *control fingers* to hold and keep the tension on the braid.

Also, it is very important to work on twisting your wrists to create the motion and tension required. Keep your wrists loose and flexible. Your wrist movements help to maintain tension and correct positioning of the strands of hair.

Braid to End

Your braid should be even all the way to the end. You should practice this braid until doing it is easy – left under middle, right under middle, left under middle, right under middle.

Next Practice Braid

Now, reduce the size of your braid. Make a square that is about 1" by 1". Divide this section into three equal parts. Then braid – left under middle – right under middle.

Do this braid over and over until you feel comfortable with the finger and wrist movements. When you feel comfortable braiding and your braid is neat and even – from the roots to the end of the braid – you can move on to the next type of braid.

UNDER FILLER FIBER BRAID

Introduction

This is called an under filler fiber braid because you will be using a filler fiber to create an under braid. You will always be moving one section of the three sections under the middle section. This is the same as the under braid you just learned, except one strand will be the hair from the Manikin and two strands will be filler fiber.

Set up your Manikin facing away from you.

Hands, Fingers and Wrists

Working Fingers
These fingers are called your working fingers. They will manipulate the hair to be moved.

Control Fingers
These fingers are referred to as your control fingers because they control the hair – holding it in place and maintaining tension as you are braiding.

Wrist Movement
Keep your wrists loose and flexible. Your wrist movements are important in helping to maintain tension, in correct positioning of the strands of hair and in the total appearance of the braid.

Prepare Filler Fiber

Filler fiber is any synthetic fiber that has an extremely tight curl. You will always use the same thickness of filler fiber as you are using of natural hair. In this case, for your first practice braid, you will need about 1" thick strand. The length of the filler fiber will depend on how long your braid will be. Since you will be braiding hair that is 8" long, you need fiber that is about 16-20" long – double the length of the braid you are creating.

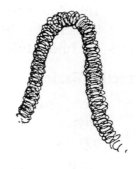

Trim the ends so that they are neat and won't tangle while you are braiding. To make the fiber more manageable, it is helpful to spray it with water or hair spray.

BRAIDING AND SEWING TRACKS

Make a Square

For your first practice under filler fiber braid, take a 1" square section of hair at the center front of the hairline on your Manikin. In your left hand, hold the hair straight up from the Manikin's head.

Placement of Fiber

Hold the filler fiber in your right hand and loop it around the hair, creating a "V".

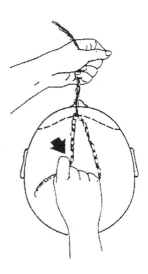

With your left hand, pull the Manikin's hair down so that it is straight out – above the Manikin's nose.

With your right palm facing down, hold the left strand of the filler fiber in between your second working finger and your first control finger.

Lock In Twist

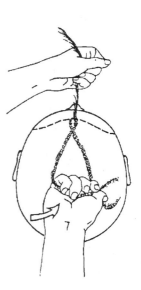

Next, turn your right hand palm up. This will cause the filler fiber to cross over. The objective is to get the filler fiber as close to the scalp as possible before proceeding with the braid.

First Cross Under

Pick Up Strand
With your left working fingers, reach under your right hand and pick up the right strand.

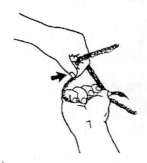

Twist Wrist
Twist your left wrist – causing your palm to face upward. This motion will pull the right strand under the center strand.

The new middle strand will now be in your left working fingers.

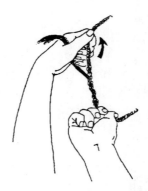

Transfer Strand
Transfer the strand in your right working fingers to your right control fingers. Maintain the tension.

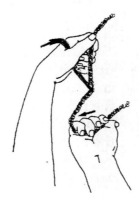

Second Cross Under

Pick Up Strand
With your right working fingers, reach under your left hand and pick up the left strand.

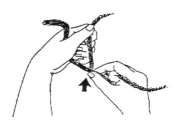

Twist Wrist
Twist your right wrist – causing your palm to face upward. This motion will pull the left strand under the center strand.

The new middle strand will now be in your right working fingers.

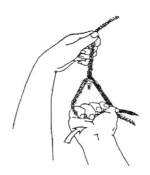

Transfer Strand
Transfer the strand in your left working fingers to your left control fingers. Maintain the tension.

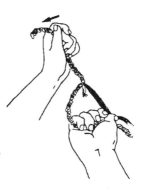

Third Cross Under

Pick Up Strand
With your left working fingers, reach under your right hand and pick up the right strand.

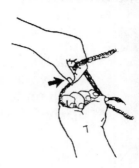

Twist Wrist
Twist your left wrist – causing your palm to face upward. This motion will pull the right strand under the center strand.

The new middle strand will now be in your left working fingers.

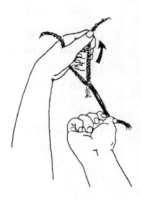

Transfer Strand
Transfer the strand in your right working fingers to your right control fingers. Maintain the tension.

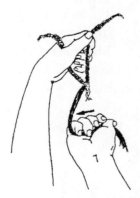

Fourth Cross Under

Pick Up Strand
With your right working fingers, reach under your left hand and pick up the left strand.

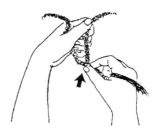

Twist Wrist
Twist your right wrist – causing your palm to face upward. This motion will pull the left strand under the center strand.

The new middle strand will now be in your right working fingers.

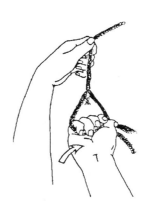

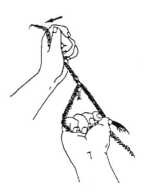

Transfer Strand
Transfer the strand in your left working fingers to your left control fingers. Maintain the tension.

Fifth Cross Under

Pick Up Strand
With your left working fingers, reach under your right hand and pick up the right strand.

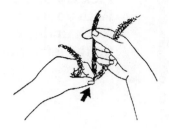

Twist Wrist
Twist your left wrist – causing your palm to face upward. This motion will pull the right strand under the center strand.

The new middle strand will now be in your left working fingers.

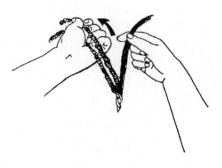

Transfer Strand
Transfer the strand in your right working fingers to your right control fingers. Maintain the tension.

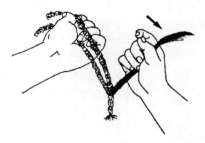

Sixth Cross Under

Pick Up Strand
With your right working fingers, reach under your left hand and pick up the left strand.

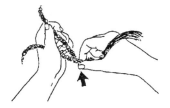

Twist Wrist
Twist your right wrist – causing your palm to face upward. This motion will pull the left strand under the center strand.

The new middle strand will now be in your right working fingers.

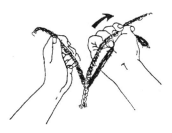

Transfer Strand
Transfer the strand in your left working fingers to your left control fingers. Maintain the tension.

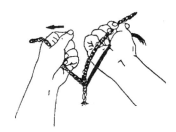

Continue Braiding

Remember to use your working fingers to pick up the hair to be moved (braided) and your control fingers to hold and keep the tension on the braid. Also, it is very important to work on twisting your wrists to create the motion and tension required.

Braid to End

Your braid should be even all the way to the end. You should practice this braid until doing it is easy – left under middle, right under middle, left under middle, right under middle.

Next Practice Braid

Now, reduce the size of your braid. Reduce the amount, the thickness of your filler fiber to 1/2". On the Manikin, make a square that is about 1/2" x 1/2" of hair. Divide this section into three equal parts. Then braid – left under middle – right under middle.

Do this braid over and over until you feel comfortable with the finger and wrist movements. When you feel comfortable braiding and your braid is neat and even – from the roots to the end of the braid – you can move on to the next type of braid.

The most important thing to work on for this braid is to try and get the filler fiber close to the scalp when you begin – and to be sure that it stays close to the scalp when you have finished the braid.

Remember the picture of the double helix in the preface. This may be a difficult task but with practice you can master it!

UNDER BRAID ON SCALP

Introduction

This is an under braid that is on the scalp because you will be picking up hair from the Manikin's head and braiding it into the three strands.

Set up your Manikin with the face away from your body.

Hands, Fingers and Wrists

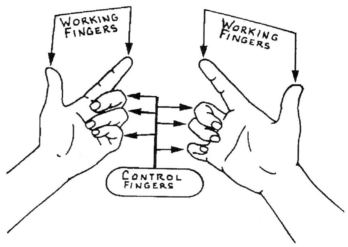

Working Fingers
These fingers are called your working fingers. They will manipulate the hair to be moved.

Control Fingers
These fingers are called your control fingers because they control the hair – holding it in place and maintaining tension as you are braiding.

Wrist Movement
Keep your wrists loose and flexible. Your wrist movements are important in helping to maintain tension, in correct positioning of the strands of hair and in the total appearance of the braid.

Make a Part

For your first practice under braid on the scalp, make a 1" wide section by parting the hair at the center front of the hair line on your Manikin. Clip down the hair that you will not be braiding.

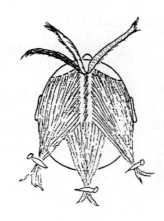

Make a Section

Make a section then divide it into three equal parts.

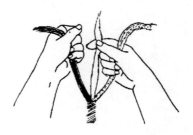

In your right hand – your right control fingers – hold the right strand.

In your right hand – your right working fingers – hold the middle strand.

In your left hand – your left control fingers – hold the left strand.

Important: You will be using your working fingers a lot. They move the strands through the braid and they pick up the hair.

First Cross Under

Pick Up Strand
Twist your left wrist – causing your palm to face upward

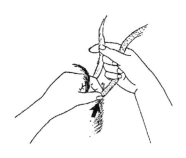

Twist Wrist
Twist your left wrist – causing your palm to face upward. This motion will pull the right strand under the center strand.

The new middle strand will now be in your left working fingers.

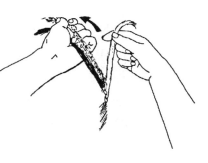

Transfer Strand
Transfer the strand in your right working fingers to your right control fingers. Maintain the tension.

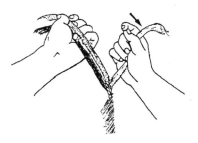

Second Cross Under

Pick Up Strand
With your right working fingers, reach under your left hand and pick up the left strand.

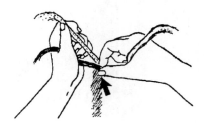

Twist Wrist
Twist your right wrist – causing your palm to face upward. This motion will pull the left strand under the center strand.

The new middle strand will now be in your right working fingers.

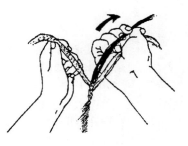

Transfer Strand
Transfer the strand in your left working fingers to your left control fingers. Maintain the tension.

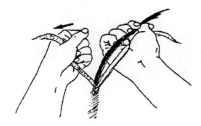

Third Cross Under

Pick Up Strand
With your left working fingers, reach under your right hand and pick up the right strand.

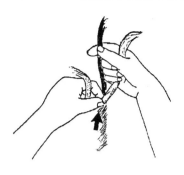

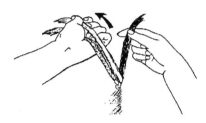

Twist Wrist
Twist your left wrist – causing your palm to face upward. This motion will pull the right strand under the center strand.

The new middle strand will now be in your left working fingers.

Transfer Strand
Transfer the strand in your right working fingers to your right control fingers. Maintain the tension.

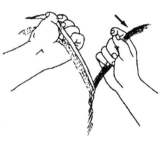

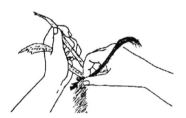

Pick Up Scalp Hair
With your right working fingers, pick up hair from the part.

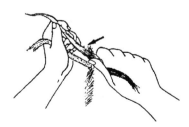

Add To Center Strand
Add this hair to the center strand which is in your left working fingers.

Fourth Cross Under

Pick Up Strand
Pick up the left strand.

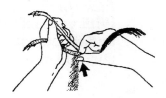

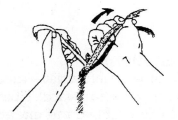

Twist Wrist
Twist your right wrist – causing your palm to face upward. This motion will pull the left strand under the center strand.

The new middle strand will now be in your right working fingers.

Transfer Strand
Transfer the strand in your left working fingers to your left control fingers. Maintain the tension.

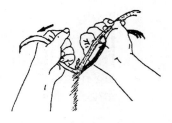

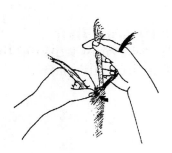

Pick Up Scalp Hair
With your left working fingers, pick up hair from the part.

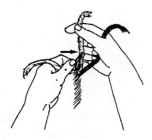

Add To Center Strand
Add this hair to the center strand which is in your right working fingers.

Fifth Cross Under

Pick Up Strand
With your left working fingers, reach under your right hand and pick up the right strand.

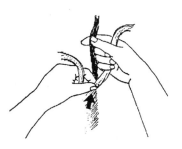

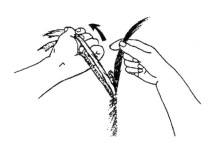

Twist Wrist
Twist your left wrist – causing your palm to face upward. This motion will pull the right strand under the center strand.

The new middle strand will now be in your left working fingers.

Transfer Strand
Transfer the strand in your right working fingers to your right control fingers. Maintain the tension.

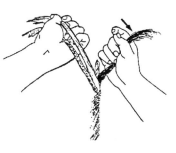

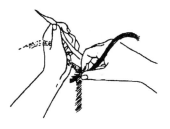

Pick Up Scalp Hair
With your right working fingers, pick up hair from the part.

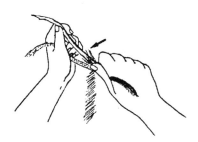

Add To Center Strand
Add this hair to the center strand which is in your left working fingers.

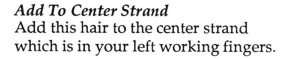

Sixth Cross Under

Pick Up Strand
With your right working fingers, reach under your left hand and pick up the left strand.

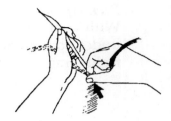

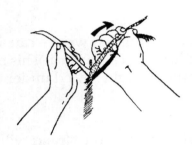

Twist Wrist
Twist your right wrist – causing your palm to face upward. This motion will pull the left strand under the center strand.

The new middle strand will now be in your right working fingers.

Transfer Strand
Transfer the strand in your left working fingers to your left control fingers. Maintain the tension.

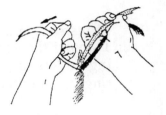

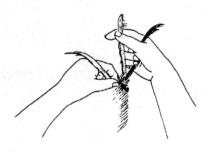

Pick Up Scalp Hair
With your left working fingers, pick up hair from the part.

Add To Center Strand
Add this hair to the center strand which is in your right working fingers.

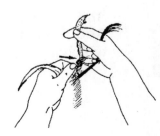

Continue Braiding

To help keep your tension, push the Manikin head forward.

Remember to use your working fingers to pick up the hair to be moved (braided or added to the braid) and your control fingers to hold and keep the tension on the braid. Also, it is very important to work on twisting your wrists to create the motion and tension required.

Braid to End

Your braid should be even all the way to the end. You should practice this braid until doing it is easy – left under middle, right under middle, left under middle, right under middle.

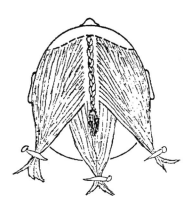

Next Practice Braid

Now, reduce the size of your braid. Make a part that is about 1/2" wide. Divide this section into three equal parts then braid.

Do this braid over and over until you feel comfortable with the finger and wrist movements. When you feel comfortable braiding and your braid is neat and even (from the begining to the end of the part) and the parting is clean (no hairs from outside the part are captured in the braid) you can move on to the next type of braid.

UNDER FILLER FIBER BRAID ON SCALP

Introduction

This is called an under filler fiber braid on the scalp because you will be using a filler fiber to create an under braid and you will be adding hair from the scalp. You will always be moving one section of the three sections under the middle section. This is the same as the under braid on scalp that you just learned, except you will be using one strand of hair from the Manikin and two strands will be filler fiber.

This is the practice braid that will help you to do tracking of what are called micro filler fiber braids that are used for the Braid and Sew attachment technique.

Set up your Manikin facing away from you.

Hands, Fingers and Wrists

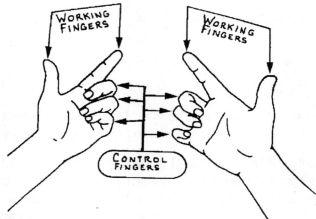

Working Fingers
These fingers are called your working fingers. They will manipulate the hair to be moved.

Control Fingers
These fingers are referred to as your control fingers because they control the hair – holding it in place and maintaining tension as you are braiding.

Wrist Movement
Keep your wrists loose and flexible. Your wrist movements are important in helping to maintain tension, in correct positioning of the strands of hair and in the total appearance of the braid.

Prepare Filler Fiber

Remember, You will always use the same thickness of filler fiber as you are using of natural hair. In this case, for your first practice braid, you will need about 1" thick strand. The length of the filler fiber will depend on how long your braid will be. Since you will be creating a braid that is about 6" long, you will need about 14" of fiber — double the length of the braid you are creating.

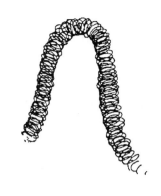

Trim the ends so that they are neat and won't tangle on you while you are braiding. To make the fiber more manageable, it is helpful to spray it with water or hair spray.

Make a Part

For your first practice braid, make a 1" wide parting. Part the hair at the center front of the hairline on your Manikin. Clip down the hair that you will not be braiding.

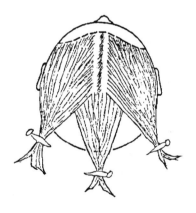

Make a Section

Take one section of hair, the width of the part, in your left hand. Hold this section straight up from the Manikin's head.

Placement of Fiber

Hold the filler fiber in your right hand and loop it around the hair, creating a "V".

With your left hand, pull the Manikin's hair down so that it is straight out – above the Manikin's nose.

With your right palm facing down, hold the left strand of the filler fiber in between your second working finger and your first control finger.

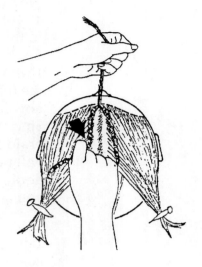

Lock In Twist

Turn your right hand palm up. This will cause the filler fiber to cross over. The objective is to get the filler fiber as close to the scalp as possible before proceeding with the braid.

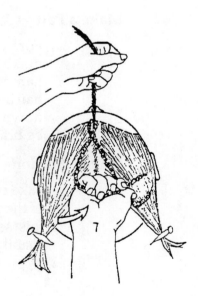

BRAIDING AND SEWING TRACKS

First Cross Under

Pick Up Strand
You will be doing two cross unders before you pick up hair from the scalp and add to the center strand. This is because you want to "lock in" the filler fiber – to get it as close to the scalp as possible before proceeding with the braid.

With your left working fingers, reach under your right hand and pick up the right strand.

Twist Wrist
Twist your left wrist – causing your palm to face upward. This motion will pull the right strand under the center strand.

The new middle strand will now be in your left working fingers.

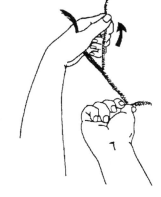

Transfer Strand
PX121

Transfer the strand in your right working fingers to your right control fingers. Maintain the tension.

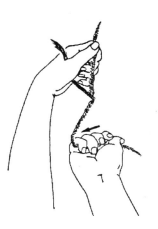

Second Cross Under

Pick Up Strand
With your right working fingers, reach under your left hand and pick up the left strand.

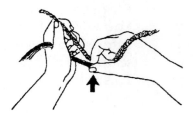

Twist Wrist
Twist your right wrist – causing your palm to face upward. This motion will pull the left strand under the center strand.

The new middle strand will now be in your right working fingers.

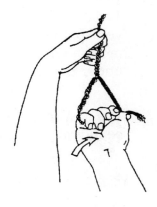

Transfer Strand
Transfer the strand in your left working fingers to your left control fingers. Maintain the tension.

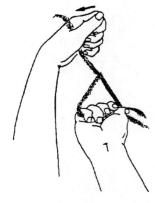

Third Cross Under

Pick Up Strand
With your left working fingers, reach under your right hand and pick up the right strand.

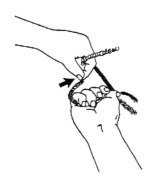

Twist Wrist
Twist your left wrist – causing your palm to face upward. This motion will pull the right strand under the center strand.

The new middle strand will now be in your left working fingers.

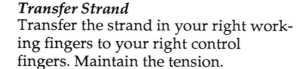

Transfer Strand
Transfer the strand in your right working fingers to your right control fingers. Maintain the tension.

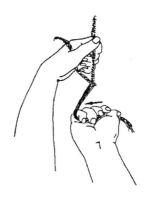

Pick Up Scalp Hair
With your right working fingers, pick up hair from the part.

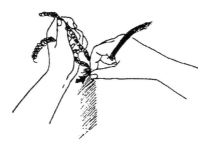

Add To Center Strand
Add this hair to the center strand which is in your left working fingers.

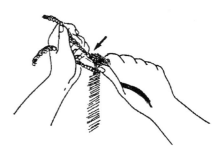

Fourth Cross Under

Pick Up Strand
With your right working fingers, reach under your left hand and pick up the left strand.

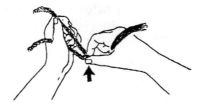

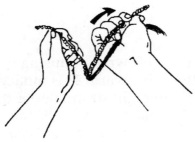

Twist Wrist
Twist your right wrist – causing your palm to face upward. This motion will pull the left strand under the center strand.

The new middle strand will now be in your right working fingers.

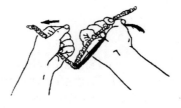

Transfer Strand
Transfer the strand in your left working fingers to your left control fingers. Maintain the tension.

Pick Up Scalp Hair
With your left working fingers, pick up hair from the part.

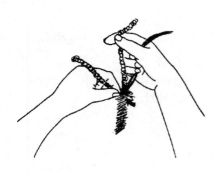

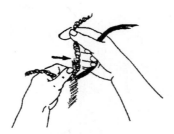

Add To Center Strand
Add this hair to the center strand which is in your right working fingers.

BRAIDING AND SEWING TRACKS

Fifth Cross Under

Pick Up Strand
With your left working fingers, reach under your right hand and pick up the right strand.

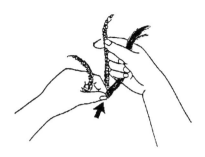

Twist Wrist
Twist your left wrist – causing your palm to face upward. This motion will pull the right strand under the center strand.

The new middle strand will now be in your left working fingers.

Transfer Strand
Transfer the strand in your right working fingers to your right control fingers. Maintain the tension.

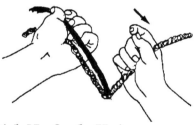

Pick Up Scalp Hair
With your right working fingers, pick up hair from the part.

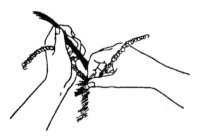

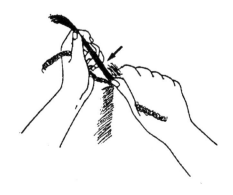

Add To Center Strand
Add this hair to the center strand which is in your left working fingers.

Sixth Cross Under

Pick Up Strand
With your right working fingers, reach under your left hand and pick up the left strand.

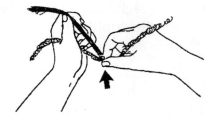

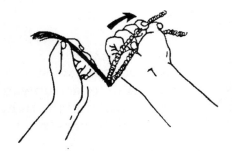

Twist Wrist
Twist your right wrist – causing your palm to face upward. This motion will pull the left strand under the center strand.

The new middle strand will now be in your right working fingers.

Transfer Strand
Transfer the strand in your left working fingers to your left control fingers. Maintain the tension.

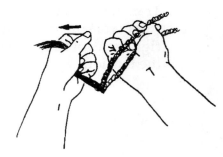

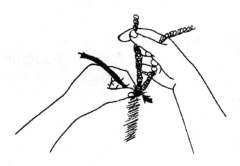

Pick Up Scalp Hair
With your left working fingers, pick up hair from the part.

Add To Center Strand
Add this hair to the center strand which is in your right working fingers.

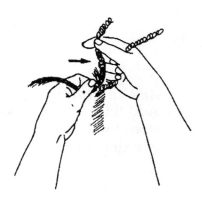

Continue Braiding

Remember to use your working fingers to pick up the hair to be moved (braided) and your control fingers to hold and keep the tension on the braid. Also, it is very important to work on twisting your wrists to create the motion and tension required.

Braid to End

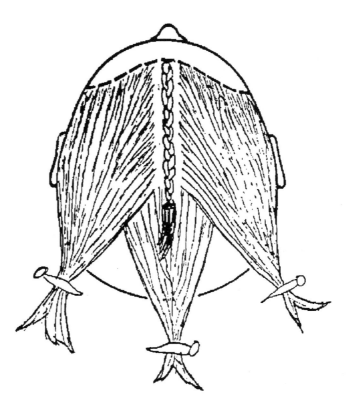

Your braid should be even all the way to the end. You should practice this braid until doing it is easy – left under middle, right under middle, left under middle, right under middle.

Next Practice Braid

Now, reduce the size of your braid. Make a part that is about 1/2" wide and the filler fiber will be 1/2" thick.

Do this braid over and over until you feel comfortable with the finger and wrist movements. When you feel comfortable braiding and your braid is neat and even (from the roots to the end of the braid), and the part is clean (no hairs outside of the part are captured in the braid), you can move on to making tracks.

MAKING BRAIDED TRACKS

Introduction

A braided track is a micro filler fiber braid (is the same as an under filler fiber braid on the scalp). This braid is like the braid you learned before, except that you will be braiding horizontally rather than vertically.

To make a braided track, you will make two braids, one from the right and one from the left side of your Manikin's head – meeting in the center of the Manikin's head.

Set up your Manikin with its right ear facing your body. Use a water bottle and slightly wet the hair on the Manikin before making your part.

Sectioning Hair for Tracking

Now you are ready to section the hair on your Manikin in preparation for making a track.

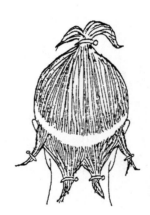

In Chapter 8 *Putting It All Together* you will learn more about exact placement for tracks relative to designing the style. For right now you are going to learn about the basics.

You will make a track using 1/4" to 1/2" of hair.

For hair that is **thick,** you will make your part 1/4" wide.

For hair that is thin, you will make your part 1/2" wide.

You always begin your sections at the bottom of your style, usually 1" above hairline at the nape of the neck. You build a style from the bottom up – like building a house – from the bottom up.

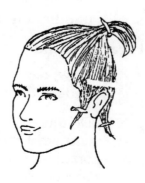

You will usually leave 1/2" to 1" of hair loose on either side of the track. This loose hair will cover (hide) the track.

Make a clean U-shaped part. A clean part is very, very important. Be sure you secure the loose hair, above and below the part. Any loose hair that becomes a part of the braid is painful for your client and that hair will eventually end up being pulled out of the scalp.

For practice on your first track you do not need to be concerned with the placement of the track. Make your practice track in about the middle of your Manikin's head so you can concentrate on mastering the braiding.

Hands, Fingers and Wrists

Working Fingers
These fingers are called your working fingers. They will manipulate the hair to be moved.

Control Fingers
These fingers are called your control fingers because they control the hair – holding it in place and maintaining tension as you are braiding.

Wrist Movement
Keep your wrists loose and flexible. Your wrist movements are important in helping to maintain tension, in correct positioning of the strands of hair and in the total appearance of the braid.

Prepare Filler Fiber

You will always use the same thickness of filler fiber as you are using of natural hair. In this case, you will need 1/2" to 1/4" thick strand (depending on the width of your parting on the Manikin). The length of the filler fiber will about 14-16".

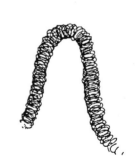

Trim the ends so that they are neat and won't tangle while you are braiding. To make the fiber more manageable, it is helpful to spray it with water or hair spray.

Placement of Fiber

Take one section of hair, the width of the part and in your left hand, hold the hair straight, as shown.

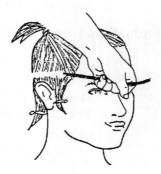

Hold the filler fiber in your right hand and loop it around the hair, creating a "V".

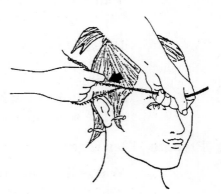

With your right palm facing down, hold the left strand of the filler fiber in between your second working finger and your first control finger.

Lock In Twist

Next, turn your right hand palm up. This will cause the filler fiber to cross over. The objective is to get the filler fiber as close to the scalp as possible before proceeding with the braid.

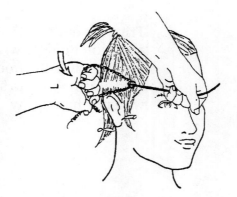

First Cross Under

Pick Up Strand

You will be doing two cross unders before you pick up hair from the scalp and add to the center strand. This is because you want to "lock in" the filler fiber – to get it as close to the scalp as possible before proceeding with the braid.

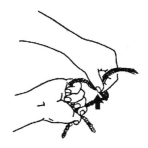

With your left working fingers, reach under your right hand and pick up the right strand.

Twist Wrist

Twist your left wrist – causing your palm to face upward. This motion will pull the right strand under the center strand.

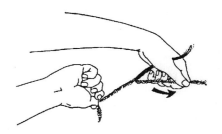

The new middle strand will now be in your left working fingers.

Transfer Strand

Transfer the strand in your right working fingers to your right control fingers. Maintain the tension.

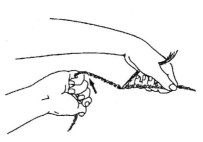

Second Cross Under

Pick Up Strand
With your right working fingers, reach under your left hand and pick up the left strand.

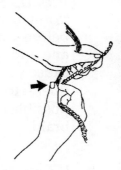

Twist Wrist
Twist your right wrist – causing your palm to face upward. This motion will pull the left strand under the center strand.

The new middle strand will now be in your right working fingers.

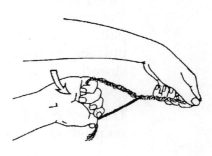

Transfer Strand
Transfer the strand in your left working fingers to your left control fingers. Maintain the tension.

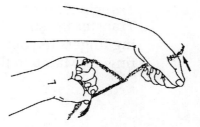

BRAIDING AND SEWING TRACKS

Third Cross Under

Pick Up Strand
With your left working fingers, reach under your right hand and pick up the right strand.

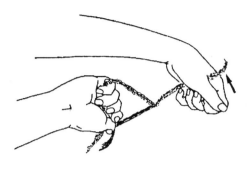

Twist Wrist
Twist your left wrist – causing your palm to face upward. This motion will pull the right strand under the center strand.

The new middle strand will now be in your left working fingers.

Transfer Strand
Transfer the strand in your right working fingers to your right control fingers. Maintain the tension.

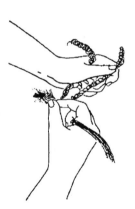

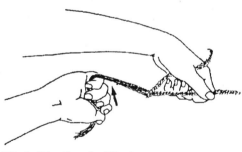

Pick Up Scalp Hair
With your right working fingers, pick up hair from the part.

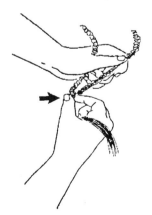

Add To Center Strand
Add this hair to the center strand which is in your left working fingers.

Fourth Cross Under

Pick Up Strand
With your right working fingers, reach under your left hand and pick up the left strand.

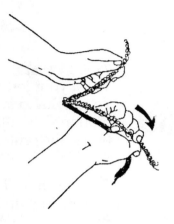

Twist Wrist
Twist your right wrist – causing your palm to face upward. This motion will pull the left strand under the center strand.

The new middle strand will now be in your right working fingers.

Transfer Strand
Transfer the strand in your left working fingers to your left control fingers. Maintain the tension.

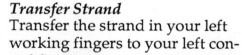

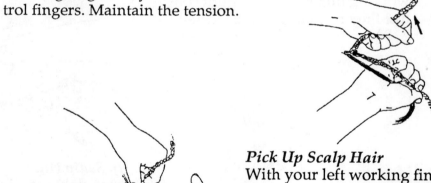

Pick Up Scalp Hair
With your left working fingers, pick up hair from the part.

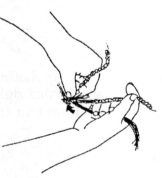

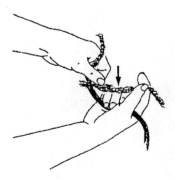

Add To Center Strand
Add this hair to the center strand which is in your right working fingers.

BRAIDING AND SEWING TRACKS

Fifth Cross Under

Pick Up Strand
With your left working fingers, reach under your right hand and pick up the right strand.

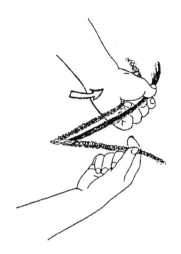

Twist Wrist
Twist your left wrist – causing your palm to face upward. This motion will pull the right strand under the center strand.

The new middle strand will now be in your left working fingers.

Transfer Strand
Transfer the strand in your right working fingers to your right control fingers. Maintain the tension.

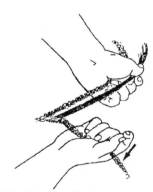

Pick Up Scalp Hair
With your right working fingers, pick up hair from the part.

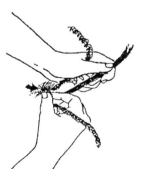

Add To Center Strand
Add this hair to the center strand which is in your left working fingers.

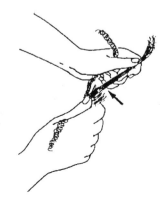

Sixth Cross Under

Pick Up Strand
With your right working fingers, reach under your left hand and pick up the left strand.

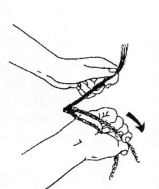

Twist Wrist
Twist your right wrist – causing your palm to face upward. This motion will pull the left strand under the center strand.

The new middle strand will now be in your right working fingers.

Transfer Strand
Transfer the strand in your left working fingers to your left control fingers. Maintain the tension.

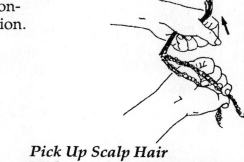

Pick Up Scalp Hair
With your left working fingers, pick up hair from the part.

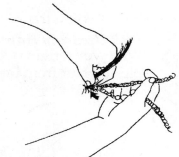

Add To Center Strand
Add this hair to the center strand which is in your right working fingers.

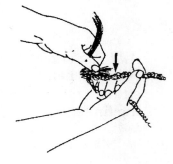

Continue Braiding

To help keep your tension, push the Manikin head away from your body. Remember to use your working fingers to pick up the hair to be moved (braided) and your control fingers to hold and keep the tension on the braid. Also, it is very important to work on twisting your wrists to create the motion and tension required.

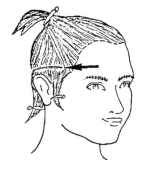

Most important – make sure your braid is started correctly. At the beginning of the braid (see the arrow), if the filler fiber slips, then there will be drag – too much stress on the hair. This is where baldness can occur **if** the braid is not done correctly. On your clients, be sure to check this area regularly. Look for redness of the scalp. Any redness should disappear after a day or two. If any redness on the scalp continues, the braid may be too tight or there may be too much drag/stress in the area where there is redness. Also, some clients have "hot spots." These are areas where their scalp is exceptionally sensititive. You may need to avoid these areas.

Braid to the Middle of the Head

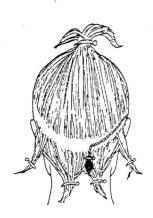

Your braid should be even all the way – sitting flat against the head. You can temporarily finish this braid off by putting a clip or by wrapping a rubber band at the end of the braid. (Later in this chapter you'll learn about different ways to finish off a track.)

Begin Other Side of the Track

Now begin another braid at the other side of the head. Braid the same way as you did on the first side.

Check Braid

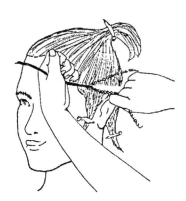

Now, look at both of your braids. Are they looser and wider at the center than they are when you started? If so, before you move on – do this braid again and again until it is the same size (thickness and tightness) all the way to the end of the braid.

Follow Curvature of the Head

The secret of correct placement of tracks is to follow the curvature of your client's head. Besides insuring correct placement of the track you will be able to better control the tension of the braid.

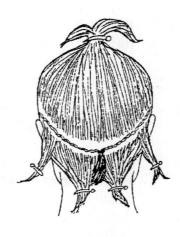

Avoid working in awkward positions. Doing what comes naturally works. By this I mean, move your body in addition to moving your Manikin's (client's) head.

Correct Tension

Correct tension on the braid is important. If the braid is too loose, when the weft is sewn on, the weight of the weft will pull the braid away from the scalp. A braid that drags can cause damage to the hair, particularly delicate hair. A braid that is too tight is also a hazard. People who are used to having their hair braided are used to the "pain" and may not feel any discomfort. However, the discomfort is not the main hazard. It is the damage to the client's scalp and hair that can be serious. The scalp should not pull away from the head. Watch for a rash that may develop on your client. Also, some clients have "hot spots" which you may need to avoid.

Keep the Braid CLEAN

Neat clean parts are the first step for a clean braid. Always watch for loose hairs as you are braiding. Any loose hairs caught in the braid will be painful (for the client). And, chances are, the hair will pull out due to tension.

Practice, Practice, Practice

Practice this braid as many times as you need to – until you can do it automatically and the braid is consistent in size and tension.

Major Problems

The biggest problem, the most difficult task, is getting the braid *started* correctly. The filler fiber must be at the very beginning of the braid. It is at this point that often there is too much stress on the roots of the hair. If the braid is not done correctly, "hot spots" and even bald spots can occur.

Another problem is keeping the tension consistent. The only way to master this braid is to practice and practice and practice. You'll get cramps in your fingers, you'll get frustrated – but I guarantee, with practice you can do it!

FINISHING OFF TRACKS

Introduction

When doing U-shaped tracking at the back of the head, two braids per track are recommended for several reasons. The first reason is that two braids distribute the hair at the end of the braid at the back of the head – rather than creating a large bulky "bump" on one side or the other. Also the two-braid track helps you to make neater, tension correct braids – rather than one long braid.

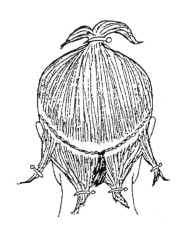

Ponytail Finish

If the track is done on thick hair and the track is thick, (that is to say, the track will easily carry the weight of the weft) you should do the ponytail finish.

After you have created two braids, you'll incorporate these two braids into one, at the center of the head.

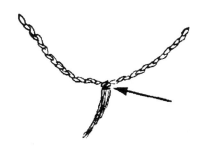

Take the hair from the ends of both braids and make into one section. Divide this section into three equal parts. Then braid these three parts only a few times.

At the end of this short braid, wrap a rubber band around the end, which should still be fairly close to the scalp. (The rubber band will remain on the head.)

You now have a small ponytail at the middle of the head which will be covered by the weft.

Braided Support Finish

If the track is thin and/or you feel that the hair on the client's scalp may be stressed by the weight of the weft, then you should do the braided support finish.

This is done by braiding the hair on each braid all the way to the end of the braid.

Secure the end of each braid with a rubber band, which will remain on the head.

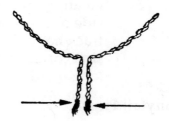

Next, cross over the braid onto the track. The braid will be secured by sewing it to the track.

To sew it you will use a large needle and cotton covered polyester thread. (See the next section on sewing for information on the needle and thread.)

Using a lock-stitch, you sew the end of the braid of one side onto the braid on the other side.

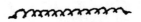

ATTACHING WEFTS TO TRACKS

Introduction

When you are doing hair extensions on a client, you will prepare the wefts before attachment. You may perm them and/or color them. However, for the sake of practice, at this point you will go ahead and attach the weft before any services are done to it.

Select Your Needle

At your local fabric store you can purchase a 7-needle set that is designed for sewing everything from sacks to sails. Among these there are two that are the best to use. These are the ones used for yarn crafts or for sacks and string sewing. Some stylists like to use a curved needle. However, control of your stitches and placement of the needle are not as good with a curved needle as it is with a straight needle.

If the point of the needle is extra sharp, file it down with a nail file or emery board.

Thread

There is only one type of thread to use – cotton covered polyester thread. 100% cotton thread will shrink when wet and dried so it should not be used. 100% polyester thread will cut through hair and because of this should not be used.

As a result, cotton covered polyester thread is the answer. The cotton protects the hair and the polyester core keeps the thread from shrinking or stretching. Also, cotton covered polyester thread dries quickly.

Measure the Width of The Weft

First, you need to determine how much of the weft you will need on each track. You do this by holding the weft up to the track.

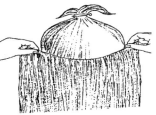

Cut the Weft

Using your working shears, cut the weft to 1/4" to 1/2" more than you will need. You don't want to come out short. If you are going to make the extension double density (thickness), cut both at the same time.

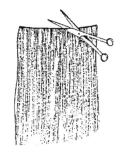

Prepare Needle, Thread and Weft

Thread the Needle
Double thread the needle and be sure to take enough thread to be able to sew the entire weft. Cut the thread from the spool and make a double knot at the end. Cut off any extra thread at the end of the knot.

For your practice sewing use a different color thread than the weft you are sewing onto the track. (Blonde thread on a dark weft.) This will make it easier for you see your work.

Needle Through Right Edge of Weft
Put the needle through the right corner of the weft, through the bottom of the stitching on the top. Pull the thread through until the knot is close to the edge of the weft.

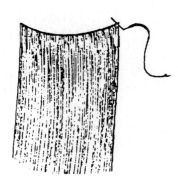

Through Loop
Next, sew through the corner of the weft to create a loop.

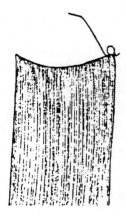

Secure Beginning
To secure the beginning of the sewing, place the needle through the loop and pull tight.

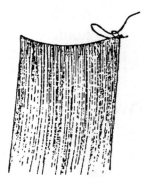

Sewing First Weft on Track

Begin at the Bottom of Braid
If you are doing two wefts per track – double density, you will sew the first weft on the bottom of the braid.

Begin by placing the weft at the right corner of the track. Put your needle through the weft, just below the stitching. Place your left forefinger above the track as a guide for your needle and as protection for your client's scalp. Then pull the needle through the weft and the bottom of the braid.

Note for left handed people: You may reverse the directions given here. In other words, you may start on the left side of the track.

Make Loop
Bring the needle around to the front. Pull it through the weft and braid until the thread makes a slight loop above the track.

Put your needle through the loop, then pull tight.

Continue Sewing
Move your needle over 3/4" of an inch for each stitch. Push the needle up – under the stitching on the weft, through or behind the braid.

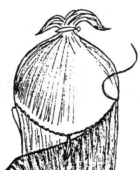

Don't Over-Sew
Next pull the needle and thread through the loop and pull tight. The type of stitch you are making is called a lock stitch. You want to make neat stitches. They do not need to be really close together nor do you want them too far apart. Don't over-sew. That is, if done neatly and tied off correctly, the sewing will be secure. Over-sewing will increase the time required for the track to dry after shampooing. Also, over-sewing means you will have more work when you want to remove the wefts.

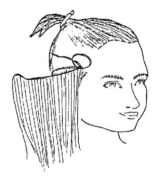

Under Ponytail
When you reach the middle of the head, if you have done a ponytail finish and you are going to put two wefts on one braid, then you will sew the first weft, the bottom weft, under the ponytail.

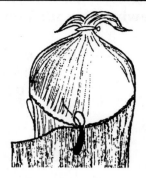

Securing at the End
At the end of the track, make a knot by going through the loop extra times. Next, cut the thread – leaving about 2-3" of extra thread. Tie a double or triple knot.

Cut off the excess thread beyond the knot.

Cut off any extra weft.

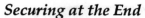

For extra security, you might want to put a drop, only a drop, of speed-bond on the knot. Remember, put the speed-bond on the knot, not the hair.

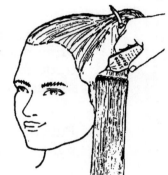

Helpful Hints
Remember to put speed-bond on the knot at the beginning of the track.

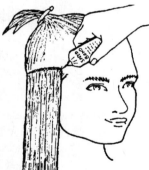

After the speed-bond has dried, be sure to check your ends and see if they are sharp. If they are, file them down with a nail file.

At the point where you have cut the weft, you may wish to place some speed-bond to keep the weft from unraveling.

While sewing, hold the weft (not yet sewn on the track) in your left control fingers, so that it won't drag.

To better manage the long thread and keep it from tangling by holding it in your left working fingers and releasing it as you sew.

If you run out of thread before you finish sewing across the entire track, make a knot, secure it with speed-bond, thread the needle and begin at the point where you stopped.

BRAIDING AND SEWING TRACKS

Sewing Second Weft on Track

Begin at Top of Braid

When you are sewing two wefts on a track, the first one goes on the bottom of the braid, whereas the second one goes on the top of the braid. However, if you are doing single-density track (only one weft per track) then you would sew that weft on the top of the track.

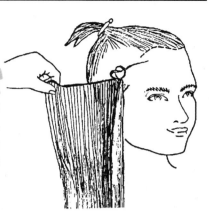

Continue Sewing

Just as you did on the bottom weft, continue sewing the weft to the braid. This time however, since you are sewing on the top of the braid, when you reach the middle, you will sew on top of the ponytail.

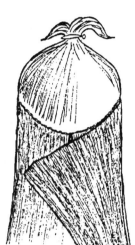

Secure at the Ends

Be sure to make multiple knots. Cut off any extra weft and secure the knots with speed-bond.

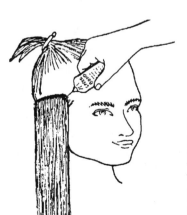
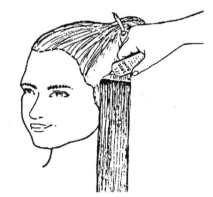

Don't forget when doing clients' hair, the speed-bond can harden on the knot and make very sharp points which can be painful for your client. Be sure to check for these and file them down with a nail file.

Also remember, make neat, clean parts. Bald spots can be caused by too much stress, by hairs that are caught in the braid from outside the part.

MAINTAINING AND RE-DOING THE STYLE

Remove Wefts

To remove this weft, simply cut the thread across the top and pull the threads out. If you have sewn the weft on correctly, this is a very simple process.

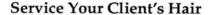

Un-Do Braids

The next step is to un-do the braids. Remember, hair that would have normally been lost (the natural shedding and replacing growth pattern) will be captured in the braid. Carefully unbraid the hair. Then brush the client's hair.

Service Your Client's Hair

A good shampoo, even a scalp massage, feels like heaven! Condition and perform any services that you may need to do to your client's hair.

Re-Do the Style

When re-doing the style, it is advisable to do the tracking in a slightly different place. Remember, it takes you almost as much time to re-do a style as it did to do the style the first time. You must charge accordingly.

SUMMARY

To learn how to do the micro filler fiber braid required for the Braid and Sew technique, it requires a great deal of practice and persistence. Because of this, it is best to practice on a Manikin.

Your hands and fingers must be positioned properly for the braid to be the proper size, location and tension. Several of *The Range of Motion* exercises described in this chapter help loosen muscles and joints, help increase efficiency, and reduce fatigue. When you get tired or frustrated – walk away for a while. *Relax*.

The Braid and Sew attachment technique is important to learn for anyone who wishes to do hair extensions. The important things to remember are: make clean parts, never let hair from outside the part be captured in the braid.

Be sure the tension is correct. When doing clients, be sure to check their scalp regularly for any redness. Too much stress on the roots of the hair can cause baldness.

Chapter 3

INDIVIDUAL BRAIDING TECHNIQUES

INTRODUCTION

Many Variations

I find this chapter a very difficult one to write. This is because there are so many different variations. One could write an entire book on individual braiding techniques.

You can add hair so that the individual braids are hidden. Or, you can add hair with the braids as a visible part of the style.

The best kind of braid to do is an over braid. The individual braiding technique I consider most important for all stylists doing hair extension services to learn is the hidden 3-strand, off the scalp braid.

Do not try to learn braiding on a person's head. You will need to practice and practice. You will need a Manikin for the hours of practice required to become proficient in doing these braids.

Selecting Locking Technique
You have three ways to secure the individual braids. They are:

- Speed-bonding
- Braid-in tie-off
- Separate tie-off

In the speed-bonding technique, you "glue" the end of the braid to secure it. This is probably the fastest but, at the same time could be hazardous. You must be neat!

In the braid-in tie-off method, you use either the hair you are adding or you add thread into the braid to secure it.

In the separate tie-off technique, you tie loose hair or fiber around the braid to secure it.

ADVANTAGES AND DISADVANTAGES

Advantages of Individual Braids

There are many different styles that can be created by using the individual braiding technique demonstrated in this book.

Advantages of Individual Braids

- The added hair will often remain on your client's head for a longer period of time.

- The hair can be added in areas where it is not possible to use other techniques.

- The client's hair will dry more quickly because there is less bulk than with a braided track and a weft.

- The client may be able to manage the style better at home in that shampooing and conditioning are easier.

- Individual braids allow for styling versatility.

- Maintenance, that is re-doing the hair extension services, can be done in shorter sessions, and only the areas that have lost hair and/or have grown out too far may need to be done.

Disadvantages of Individual Braids

- The hair that has been added, once removed, often cannot be re-used, and more hair will have to be purchased, which may increase the cost to the client.

- The client may not be able to manage the style at home because this is a more delicate attachment technique.

- This is a very time consuming service, requiring anywhere from 4 to 14 or more hours of time. As a result, if the stylist is to be paid appropriately, this technique is very expensive.

- Because of the time required to do this service, a stylist will need to work his/her book very differently.

- Because the hair may stay on a client's head longer, clients may wait too long between services, thus possibly causing undue stress and damage to their own hair.

SUPPLIES

To do individual braids you will need:

Manikin and holder
Metal tip rattail comb
Speed-bond and bond remover
Filler fiber
Cotton covered polyester thread
Nail file or manicurist's sanding block
Hand barrier cream
Shears (a "working" pair)
A weft

SPEED-BONDING TECHNIQUE

Introduction

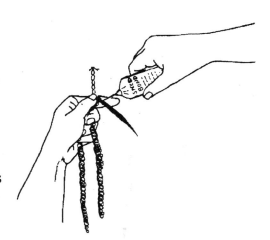

The advantage of the *speed-bonding* technique is that it is faster than the other two techniques. It also works well on all types and textures of hair.

The disadvantage, as with all individual braid techniques, is the amount of time required to do individual braids.

Prepare the Hair

As with all hair extension services, you will prepare the weft by shampooing, conditioning and, if needed, perming and/or coloring. Although you will use the hair in bunches (loose hair) rather than attached to the weft, it is better to purchase a weft rather than "bulk" hair. The reason for this is that you can perm and color the hair very easily when the hair is wefted.

Set Up Manikin

It is important to be comfortable. Set up your Manikin so that it faces away from you.

Hands and Fingers

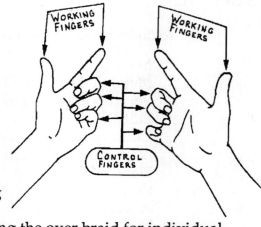

Working Fingers
These fingers are called your working fingers. They will manipulate the hair to be moved.

Control Fingers
These fingers are referred to as your control fingers because they control the hair — holding it in place and maintaining tension as you are braiding. In doing the over braid for individual braids, you will use the *1st control fingers* more *frequently* and independently from the rest of your control fingers.

Prepare Your Hands
Speed-bond will stick to your fingers. However, you can remove the build-up better if you first apply a generous amount of hand barrier cream to clean, dry fingers. You need only apply the hand barrier cream to your working fingers and 1st control finger on your left hand.

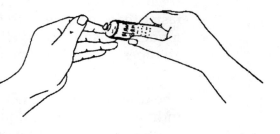

Section the Hair and Make a Square

Then, with clips, secure the hair that is not going to be braided. Section the hair according to your placement pattern. Although you will be making individual braids, following the parted "track" is very important. Make your first U-shaped part. Remember to make clean parts. Start working your style from the bottom up. For your first practice braid, take a 1/8" section of hair.

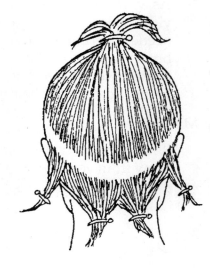

You will make the braids in a brick-layer pattern. That is, you will make a braid, then leave loose hair, braid, skip and leave loose hair, braid, then leave loose hair. Then, on your next track, you will braid above the section where you have left loose hair, and leave loose hair above the braid on the track underneath.

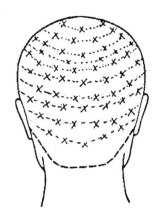

Cut the Hair

For your first speed-bond braid, you will do an equal-part fold-over braid. This means that you will be braiding an equal amount of the loose hair around the Manikin's hair.

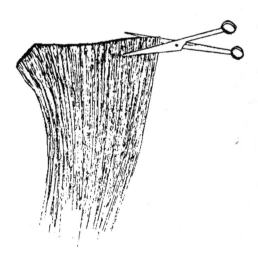

From the top of the weft, cut off approximately 1/8" of hair. This is now the loose hair you will braid into your Manikin's hair.

Your fold-over will not be exactly equal. The end that you cut from the weft should extend about 1/4" to 1/2" further than the other end. This is so you will be able to better razor cut the blunt ends in the finished style. (See Chapter 8.)

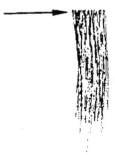

First Cross Over

Placement of Loose Hair
Place the loose hair (shown as curly) under the natural strand of hair. This is to be down, next to the scalp.

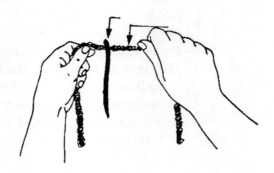

Extend Left Working Finger
Extend your left working finger, under where the loose hair and the natural hair meet.

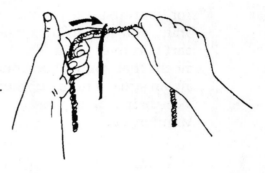

Pinch Left Working Fingers
Pinch your left working fingers together over the junction of the loose hair and the natural hair.

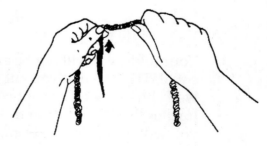

Extend Left 1st Control Finger
On your left hand, extend your 1st control finger. It will be placed in front of the natural hair strand (the middle strand).

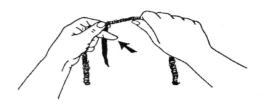

Move Right Strand Over
With your right working fingers, move the right strand over, placing it on your 1st control finger of your left hand.

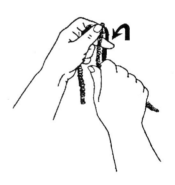

Capture Strand
Close your left control finger. The strand now is captured in your left hand and has become the center strand.

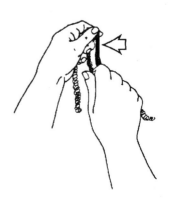

Second Cross Over

Pick Up Right Strand
With your right control fingers, pick up the right strand.

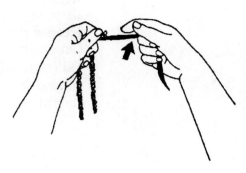

Extend Right Working Finger
Extend your right working finger and place it under the braid.

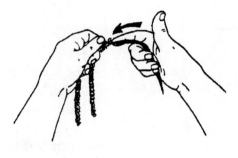

Pinch Right Working Fingers
Pinch your right working fingers together over the braid. This is how you will maintain tension on the braid.

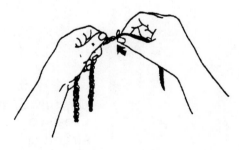

Release Center Strand
In your left control fingers, release the center strand.

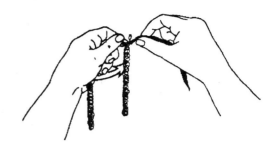

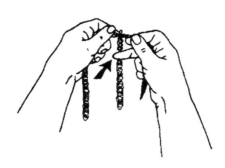

Extend Right 1st Control Finger
On your right hand, extend your 1st control finger. It will be placed in front of the middle strand.

Move Right Strand Over
With your left working fingers, move the left strand over, placing it on your 1st control finger of your right hand.

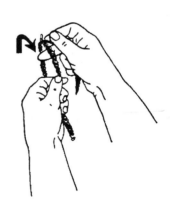

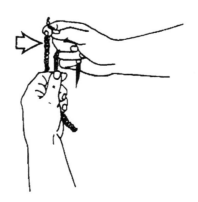

Capture Strand
Close your right control finger. The strand now is captured in your right hand and has become the center strand. Next, let go of this strand and —

Third Cross Over

Pick Up Left Strand
With your left control fingers, pick up the left strand.

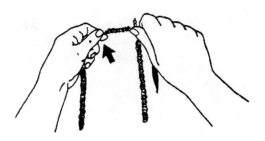

Extend Left Working Finger
Extend your left working finger and place it under the braid.

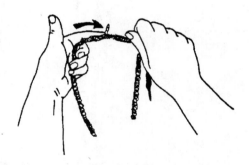

Pinch Left Working Fingers
Pinch your left working fingers together over the braid. This is how you will maintain tension on the braid.

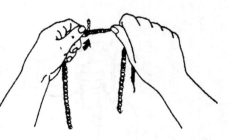

INDIVIDUAL BRAIDING TECHNIQUES

Release Center Strand
In your right control fingers, release the center strand.

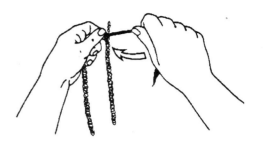

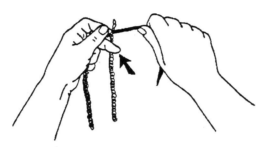

Extend Left 1st Control Finger
On your left hand, extend your 1st control finger. It will be placed in front of the middle strand.

Move Left Strand Over
With your right working fingers, move the right strand over, placing it on your 1st control finger of your left hand.

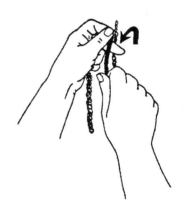

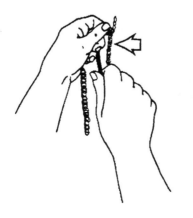

Capture Strand
Close your left control finger. The strand now is captured in your left hand and has become the center strand. Next, let go of this strand and —

Fourth Cross Over

Pick Up Right Strand
With your right control fingers, pick up the right strand.

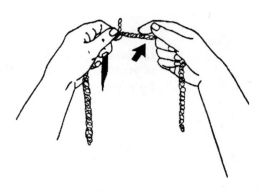

Extend Right Working Finger
Extend your right working finger and place it under the braid.

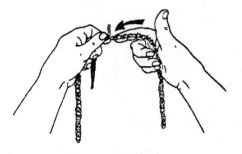

Pinch Right Working Fingers
Pinch your right working fingers together over the braid. This is how you will maintain tension on the braid.

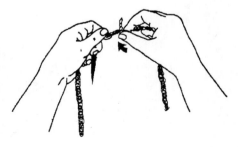

INDIVIDUAL BRAIDING TECHNIQUES

Release Center Strand
In your left control fingers, release the center strand.

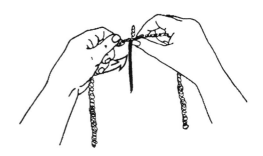

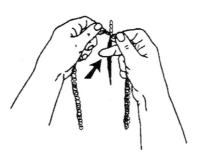

Extend Right 1st Control Finger
On your right hand, extend your 1st control finger. It will be placed in front of the middle strand.

Move Right Strand Over
With your left working fingers, move the left strand over, placing it on your 1st control finger of your right hand.

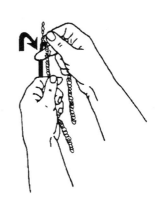

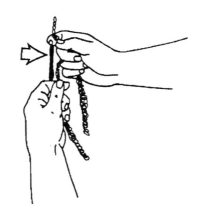

Capture Strand
Close your right control finger. The strand now is captured in your right hand and has become the center strand. Next, let go of this strand and –

Fifth Cross Over

Pick Up Left Strand
With your left control fingers, pick up the left strand.

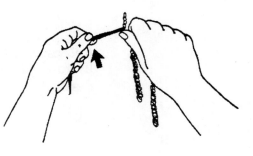

Extend Left Working Finger
Extend your left working finger and place it under the braid.

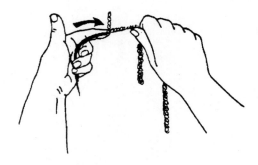

Pinch Left Working Fingers
Pinch your left working fingers together over the braid. This is how you will maintain tension on the braid.

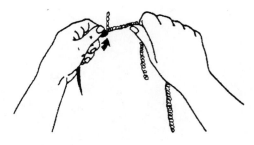

INDIVIDUAL BRAIDING TECHNIQUES

Release Center Strand
In your right control fingers, release the center strand.

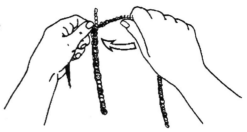

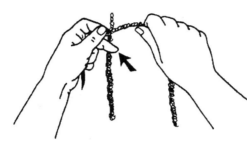

Extend Left 1st Control Finger
On your left hand, extend your 1st control finger. It will be placed in front of the middle strand.

Move Left Strand Over
With your right working fingers, move the right strand over, placing it on your 1st control finger of your left hand.

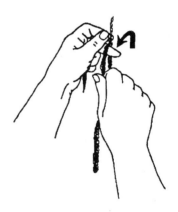

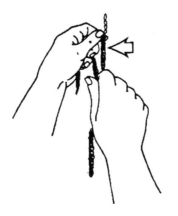

Capture Strand
Close your left control finger. The strand now is captured in your left hand and has become the center strand. Next, let go of this strand and –

Sixth Cross Over

Pick Up Right Strand
With your right control fingers, pick up the right strand.

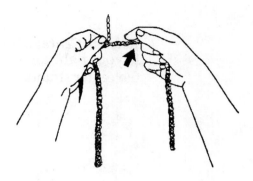

Extend Right Working Finger
Extend your right working finger and place it under the braid.

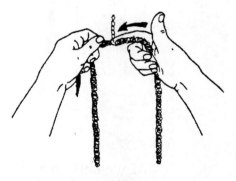

Pinch Right Working Fingers
Pinch your right working fingers together over the braid. This is how you will maintain tension on the braid.

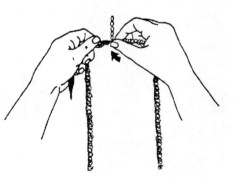

Release Center Strand
In your left control fingers, release the center strand.

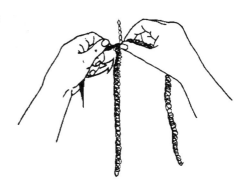

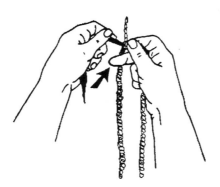

Extend Right 1st Control Finger
On your right hand, extend your 1st control finger. It will be placed in front of the middle strand.

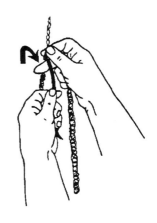

Move Right Strand Over
With your left working fingers, move the left strand over, placing it on your 1st control finger of your right hand.

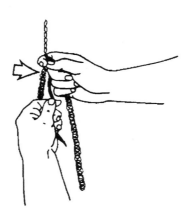

Capture Strand
Close your right control finger. The strand now is captured in your right hand and has become the center strand. Next, let go of this strand and –

Seventh Cross Over

Pick Up Left Strand
With your left control fingers, pick up the left strand.

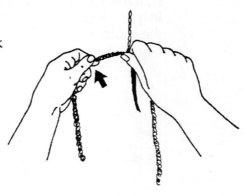

Extend Left Working Finger
Extend your left working finger and place it under the braid.

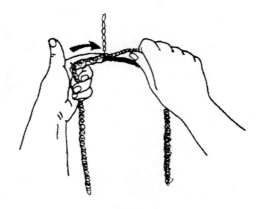

Pinch Left Working Fingers
Pinch your left working fingers together over the braid. This is how you will maintain tension on the braid.

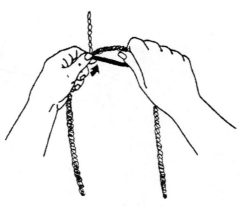

INDIVIDUAL BRAIDING TECHNIQUES

Release Center Strand
In your right control fingers, release the center strand.

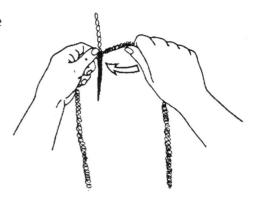

Extend Left 1st Control Finger
On your left hand, extend your 1st control finger. It will be placed in front of the middle strand.

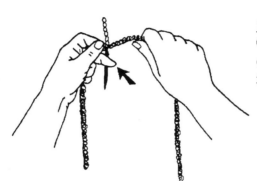

Move Left Strand Over
With your right working fingers, move the right strand over, placing it on your 1st control finger of your left hand.

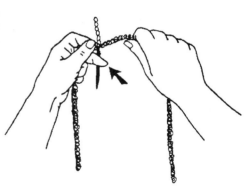

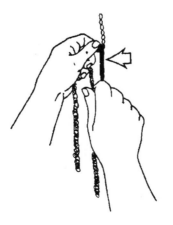

Capture Strand
Close your left control finger. The strand now is captured in your left hand and has become the center strand. Next, let go of this strand.

Reposition Braid

On curly and extremely curly hair, the braid will usually stay close to the scalp. However, on straight hair, sometimes the braid will slip away from the scalp. If this should occur, with your left thumb slide the braid back to the scalp. Be sure to maintain tension on the braid by holding the right strand (which will be the natural hair) securely in your right hand.

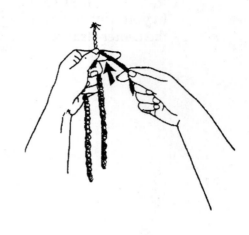

First Bonding

Hold the left and middle strands in your left control fingers. You maintain the tension by pulling on these strands. <u>With your right hand place a drop (or two) of speed-bond on the braid at the point where the middle and right strands intersect.</u>

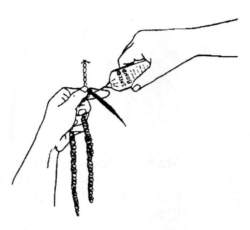

Cross Over Natural Strand

At this time, with your right hand, <u>cross the natural strand of hair over the area that has been speed-bonded.</u>

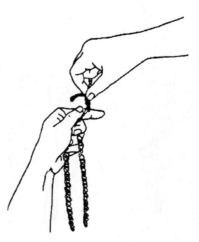

Note: These drawings show an exaggerated braid. An individual braid is actually *very small*.

INDIVIDUAL BRAIDING TECHNIQUES

Pinch Together

With your left working fingers, pinch all three strands together.

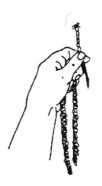

Turn Braid Over

To ensure that the end of the braid will be completely secure, turn the braid over (back side now facing you).

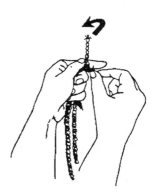

Second Bonding

At the bottom of the braid, apply one (or two) drops of speed-bond. Your objective is to apply bond carefully to both sides of the braid. It only requires a small amount of bond. Too much and the braid will be stiff and uncomfortable.

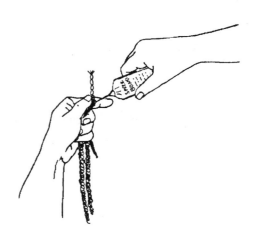

Pinch Together

After applying the speed-bond to the back side of the braid, pinch the bonded area together, using a slight side-ways movement. This will help the bond to capture all the hair.

Dealing with Finger Fatigue and Bond Build-Up

Relative to "finger fatigue", you may want to do some of the exercises explained in Chapter 2. Also, you may want to work on your client over several appointments — reducing the number of hours you are working at one time.

You will have a build-up of bond on your fingers. As you are making more braids you can use a nail file or a manicurist's sanding block to remove some of the build-up from the tips of your fingers. If you have used a hand barrier cream, the build-up will come off your fingers when you wash with soap and water. Repeat application of the barrier cream when needed.

BRAID-IN TIE-OFF WITH LOOSE HAIR TECHNIQUE

Introduction

The advantage of the braid-in tie-off with loose hair technique is that it is safer than the speed-bonding technique, particularly for a beginner.

The disadvantage, as with all individual braid techniques, is the amount of time required to do individual braids. Also, this technique does not work as well on straight and/or thin hair.

Prepare the Hair

As with all hair extension services, you will prepare the weft by shampooing, conditioning and, if needed, perming and/or coloring.

Set Up Manikin

It is important to be comfortable. Set up your Manikin so that it faces away from you.

Hands and Fingers

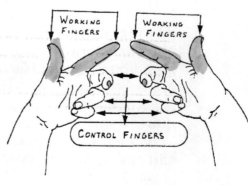

Working Fingers
These fingers are called your working fingers. They will manipulate the hair to be moved.

Control Fingers
These fingers are referred to as your control fingers because they control the hair — holding it in place and maintaining tension as you are braiding. In doing the over braid for individual braids, you will use the *1st control fingers* more *frequently* and independently from the rest of your control fingers.

INDIVIDUAL BRAIDING TECHNIQUES

Section the Hair and Make a Square

With clips, secure the hair that is not going to be braided. Section the hair according to your placement pattern. Although you will be making individual braids, following the parted "track" is very important. Make your first U-shaped part. Remember to make clean parts. Start working your style from the bottom up.

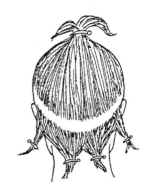

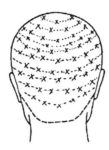

You will make the braids in a brick-layer pattern. For your first practice braid, take a 1/8" section of hair.

Cut the Hair

For this technique, you will be doing an unequal-part fold-over braid. This means that the loose hair will be longer on one side of the braid than on the other side.

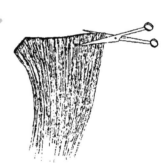

From the top of the weft, cut off approximately 1/8" hair. This is now the loose hair you will braid into your Manikin's hair.

The end that you cut from the weft will be the long side of the loose hair. This is so you will be able to better razor cut the blunt ends in the finished style. (See Chapter 8.)

Braiding Procedures

When you do the braid-in locking technique, you will fold-over the hair differently than when doing an equal fold-over as described on the preceding pages. Strand #1 (left strand) will be shorter than strand #3 (right strand). Strand #1 needs to be at least 4" of hair. Remember, have the blunt end (the end you cut from the weft) on the long side (Strand #3).

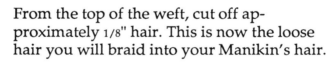

Placement of Loose Hair
Place the loose hair (shown as curly) under the natural strand of hair. This is to be down, next to the scalp.

First Cross Over

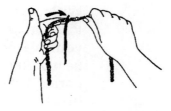

Extend: Extend your left working finger, under where the loose hair and the natural hair meet.

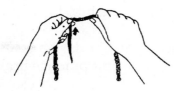

Pinch: Pinch your left working fingers together over the junction of the loose hair and the natural hair.

Extend: On your left hand, extend your 1st control finger. It will be placed in front of the natural hair strand (the middle strand).

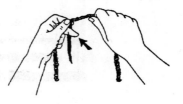

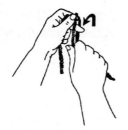

Move: With your right working fingers, move the right strand over, placing it on your 1st control finger of your left hand.

Capture: Close your left control finger. The strand now is captured in your left hand and has become the center strand.

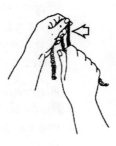

Second Cross Over

Pick Up: With your right control fingers, pick up the right strand.

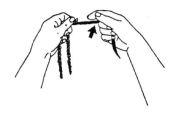

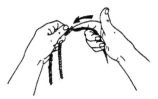

Extend: Extend your right working finger and place it under the braid.

Pinch: Pinch your right working fingers together over the braid. This is how you will maintain tension on the braid.

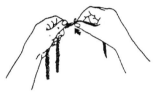

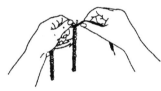

Release: In your left control fingers, release the center strand.

Extend: On your right hand, extend your 1st control finger. It will be placed in front of the middle strand.

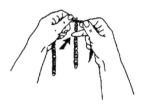

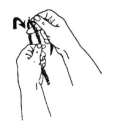

Move: With your left working fingers, move the left strand over, placing it on your 1st control finger of your right hand.

Capture: Close your right control finger. The strand now is captured in your right hand and has become the center strand. Next, let go of this strand and –

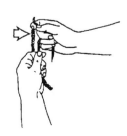

Third Cross Over

Pick Up: With your left control fingers, pick up the left strand.

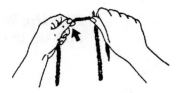

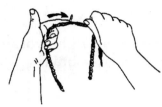

Extend: Extend your left working finger and place it under the braid.

Pinch: Pinch your left working fingers together over the braid. This is how you will maintain tension on the braid.

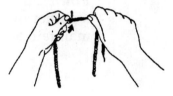

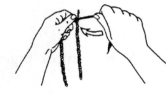

Release: In your right control fingers, release the center strand.

Extend: On your left hand, extend your 1st control finger. It will be placed in front of the middle strand.

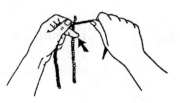

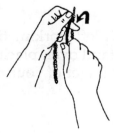

Move: With your right working fingers, move the right strand over, placing it on your 1st control finger of your left hand.

Capture: Close your left control finger. The strand now is captured in your left hand and has become the center strand. Next, let go of this strand and —

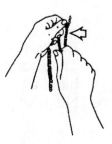

Individual Braiding Techniques

Fourth Cross Over

Pick Up: With your right control fingers, pick up the right strand.

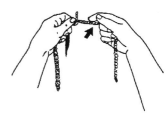

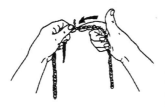

Extend: Extend your right working finger and place it under the braid.

Pinch: Pinch your right working fingers together over the braid. This is how you will maintain tension on the braid.

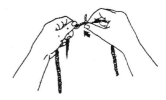

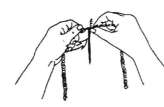

Release: In your left control fingers, release the center strand.

Extend: On your right hand, extend your 1st control finger. It will be placed in front of the middle strand.

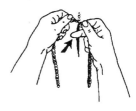

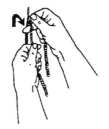

Move: With your left working fingers, move the left strand over, placing it on your 1st control finger of your right hand.

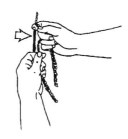

Capture: Close your right control finger. The strand now is captured in your right hand and has become the center strand. Next, let go of this strand and –

Fifth Cross Over

Pick Up: With your left control fingers, pick up the left strand.

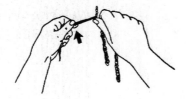

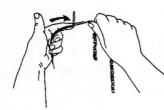

Extend: Extend your left working finger and place it under the braid.

Pinch: Pinch your left working fingers together over the braid. This is how you will maintain tension on the braid.

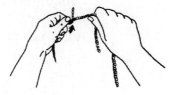

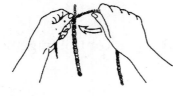

Release: In your right control fingers, release the center strand.

Extend: On your left hand, extend your 1st control finger. It will be placed in front of the middle strand.

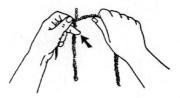

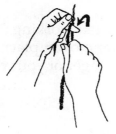

Move: With your right working fingers, move the right strand over, placing it on your 1st control finger of your left hand.

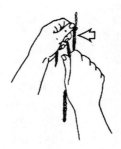

Capture: Close your left control finger. The strand now is captured in your left hand and has become the center strand. Next, let go of this strand and –

INDIVIDUAL BRAIDING TECHNIQUES

Sixth Cross Over

Pick Up: With your right control fingers, pick up the right strand.

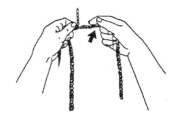

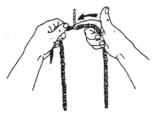

Extend: Extend your right working finger and place it under the braid.

Pinch: Pinch your right working fingers together over the braid. This is how you will maintain tension on the braid.

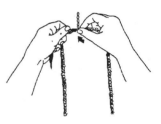

Release: In your left control fingers, release the center strand.

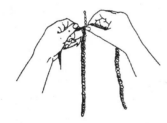

Extend: On your right hand, extend your 1st control finger. It will be placed in front of the middle strand.

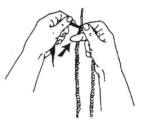

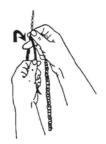

Move: With your left working fingers, move the left strand over, placing it on your 1st control finger of your right hand.

Capture: Close your right control finger. The strand now is captured in your right hand and has become the center strand. Next, let go of this strand and –

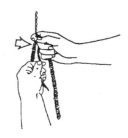

Seventh Cross Over

Pick Up: With your left control fingers, pick up the left strand.

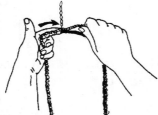

Extend: Extend your left working finger and place it under the braid.

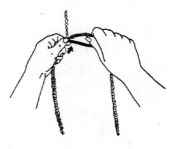

Pinch: Pinch your left working fingers together over the braid. This is how you will maintain tension on the braid.

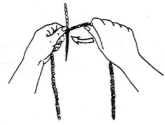

Release: In your right control fingers, release the center strand.

Extend: On your left hand, extend your 1st control finger. It will be placed in front of the middle strand.

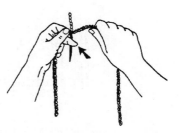

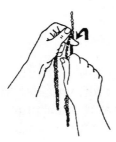

Move: With your right working fingers, move the right strand over, placing it on your 1st control finger of your left hand.

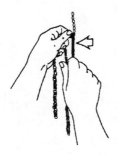

Capture: Close your left control finger. The strand now is captured in your left hand and has become the center strand. Next, let go of this strand.

INDIVIDUAL BRAIDING TECHNIQUES

Braiding Pattern Change

At this point, you will now do two more cross overs than you did for the speed-bonding technique.

Eighth Cross Over

Pick Up: With your right control fingers, pick up the right strand.

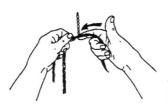

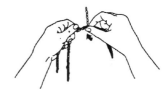

Extend: Extend your right working finger and place it under the braid.

Pinch: Pinch your right working fingers together over the braid. This is how you will maintain tension on the braid.

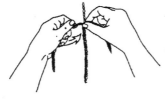

Release: In your left control fingers, release the center strand.

Extend: On your right hand, extend your 1st control finger. It will be placed in front of the middle strand.

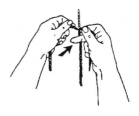

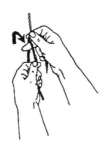

Move: With your left working fingers, move the left strand over, placing it on your 1st control finger of your right hand.

Capture: Close your right control finger. The strand now is captured in your right hand and has become the center strand. Next, let go of this strand.

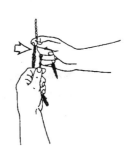

Ninth Cross Over

Pick Up: With your left control fingers, pick up the left strand.

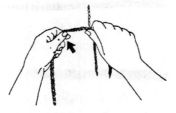

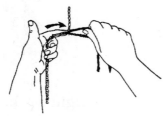

Extend: Extend your left working finger and place it under the braid.

Pinch: Pinch your left working fingers together over the braid. This is how you will maintain tension on the braid.

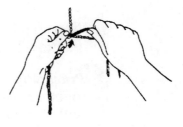

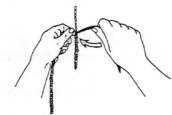

Release: In your right control fingers, release the center strand.

Extend: On your left hand, extend your 1st control finger. It will be placed in front of the middle strand.

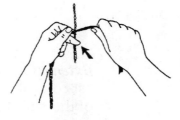

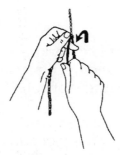

Move: With your right working fingers, move the right strand over, placing it on your 1st control finger of your left hand.

Capture: Close your left control finger. The strand now is captured in your left hand and has become the center strand. Next, let go of this strand.

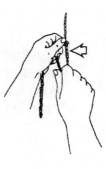

Reposition Braid: On curly and extremely curly hair, the braid will usually stay close to the scalp. However, on straight hair, sometimes the braid will slip away from the scalp. If this should occur, with your left thumb slide the braid back to the scalp. Be sure to maintain tension on the braid by holding the right strand (which will be the natural hair) securely in your right hand.

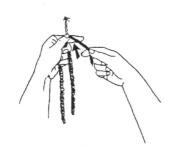

Tie-Off Procedure

Pick Up: Strand #1, the shorter strand will now be in your right hand.

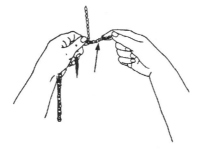

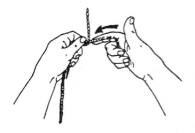

Adjust: Adjust strands in your left hand so that both are in your control fingers. Extend and place your right working finger behind the braid.

Tie Knots: Bring the right strand under, around and above the left and center strands. Next bring the strand through the loop and tighten. Repeat 2-3 more times.

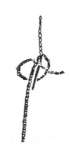

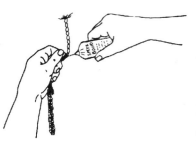

Optional: For extra security you may wish to place a drop of speed bond on the knots.

Note: These drawings show an exaggerated braid. An individual braid is actually *very small*.

BRAID-IN TIE-OFF WITH THREAD TECHNIQUE

Introduction

The advantages of the braid-in tie-off with thread technique are that it is safer than the speed-bond technique, particularly for a beginner and it is less messy. Also, compared to the braid-in tie-off with loose hair technique, it is a little easier and allows you to make smaller knots. Compare these techniques and you will see the differences in application.

The disadvantages are the same as with the other techniques already discussed. Also, this technique does not work as well on straight and/or thin hair.

Same Preparation

The preparation for this technique is the same as described previously: prepare the hair; set up the Manikin; use the same hand and fingers; section the hair and make a square; cut the hair.

Braiding Procedures

When you do the braid-in tie-off with thread technique, you can do either equal fold-over or unequal fold-over. It all depends on the finished length and density desired. (See more on this at the end of this chapter.)

Placement of Loose Hair and Thread

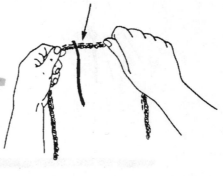

You will use about 10" of cotton covered polyester thread. Place the thread in with the loose hair. Place the loose hair (shown as curly) with the thread (shown as dots) under the natural strand of hair. This is to be down, next to the scalp.

Proceed with Braiding

Follow the instructions given for the braid-in tie-off loose hair technique – *first cross over* through *ninth cross over*.

Separate Thread

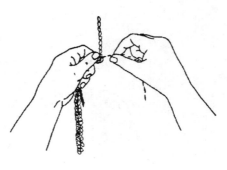

Place all three strands of the braid in your left control fingers. Separate out the thread from the hair.

INDIVIDUAL BRAIDING TECHNIQUES

Tie-Off

With your right working fingers, bring both of the threads under, around and above the braid. Then pull them through the loop and tighten. Repeat 2-3 times.

Optional

If you still want to secure the knots more, you may separate the two threads and knot them together several times. Also, you may want to place a drop of speed-bond on the knots, the threads.

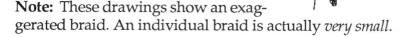

Note: These drawings show an exaggerated braid. An individual braid is actually *very small*.

SEPARATE TIE-OFF TECHNIQUE

Introduction

The tie-off locking technique works best on curly and extremely curly hair and works less well on thin, fine hair. The advantage of this locking technique over the other techniques is that it is safe for a beginner.

To tie-off the braid you can use filler fiber, thread and even loose hair.

Same Preparation

The preparation for this technique is the same as described previously: prepare the hair; set up the Manikin; use the same hand and fingers; section the hair and make a square; cut the hair.

Braiding Procedures

When you do the braid-in tie-off with thread technique, you can do either equal fold-over or unequal fold-over. It all depends on the finished length and density desired. (See more on this at the end of this chapter.)

Follow the instructions as given for the braid-in tie-off loose hair technique – *first cross over* through *ninth cross over*.

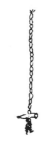

Braid Down

You will continue to braid down the strand until the braid can be held with a clip.

Tie-Off

With your working fingers, you will tie either thread, loose hair or filler fiber, close to the scalp, around the braid. Make several knots.

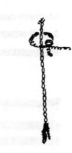

Optional

If you still want to secure the knots more, you may want to place a drop of speed-bond on the knots, the threads.

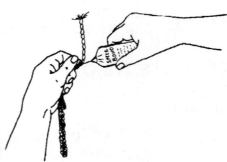

Note: These drawings show an exaggerated braid. An individual braid is actually *very small*.

DETERMINING HAIR DENSITY AND PLACEMENT

The density of the hair you are going to add will depend on how you fold-over the hair you are adding. If you do a short fold-over, the hair will be thicker at the root than at the ends. If you fold-over the hair so it is of equal parts, it will be twice as thick throughout the head.

Different fold-over lengths help you to create different styling effects. For example, if you are adding hair to the top of the head and want height, you will want a short fold-over, which, in effect, will act as a permanent back-combed area. If you are looking for a lot of volume in a specific area, such as the back of the head, you will want to do an equal part fold-over or maybe a 3/4 fold-over.

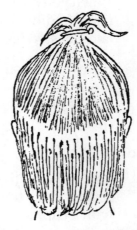

If you want long hair (longer than 10"), because of the lengths of hair available, you will have to do a 3/4 or short fold-over.

Use your imagination. Keep in mind the final style you want to create. Will the client be pulling her/his hair up or back? Which way does the client's hair naturally fall? Where are you looking for more volume, more height, more length? Don't forget to use the brick-layering technique.

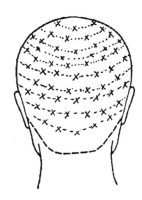

MAINTAINING AND RE-DOING THE STYLE

Removing Braids

Some individual braids will slip out on their own; others you may need to remove. It is advisable to have your client return for replacement braids on a regular basis. This should be done every 4 to 8 weeks.

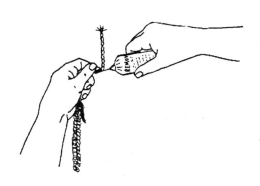

Removing braids that have been secured with knots made with thread, hair or fiber is fairly easy to do. You simply cut the knots.

Removing braids that have been secured with speed-bond requires more work. First, apply hand barrier cream to your hands. Next, apply bond remover to the bond on a braid. Then, pinch the braid with your working fingers, working the bond remover into the bond. This will soften up the speed-bond. And last, place the point of your metal-tip rattail comb at the bottom of the braid. Carefully and gently work the braid loose. Do one braid at a time.

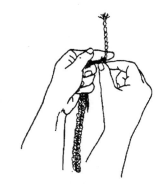

Remember, always work gently. Do not tug and pull on the hair.

Re-Doing the Style

It is recommended that you maintain any individual braid style on a regular basis. Remember, hair grows approximately 1/2" per month. The further away from the scalp the braid grows, the more stress there will be on the roots which could result in bald spots.

You may not need to remove all or even any of the braids. Sometimes you may add more hair to the section of hair that has grown out, right in front of the previous braid.

Other times you may want to add hair in other areas with or without removing the old braids. These decisions are ones you will have to make when you see your client.

SUMMARY

There are many variations of individual braiding techniques. Individually braided hair extensions have advantages and disadvantages over other techniques. These advantages and disadvantages must be considered in conjunction with each client's particular needs and home care capabilities. Because the individual braiding technique is very time consuming, you will also need to consider your bookings as they relate to your available time and to be sure that you are appropriately compensated for your skills and time.

Chapter 4

BONDING TECHNIQUES

INTRODUCTION

Definition of Bonding

Bonding hair to a client's own hair can be done several ways, using different techniques. One way is to apply a "bond" to the client's own hair and to the loose hair. The "bond" used may be a wax-type product. The method of application may be heating the "bond" with a special tool.

However, this chapter will be dedicated to the more common bonding technique. This method involves using the full weft of hair and a latex bonding material.

Not Applicable for All People

Some people can/should not have hair extensions attached by the bonding method. The reasons include:

Sensitivity to Latex (Rubber)
Some people are sensitive to the natural latex base used in adhesive bond products. These individuals are also sensitive to eyelash glues and often even adhesive bandages.

If your client is sensitive to or develops any kind of rash from latex – do not use adhesive bonds.

Extremely Damaged Hair
Some clients' hair may be severely damaged. Although one of the reasons some people have hair extensions is because they have damaged hair, you, as the stylist, may be taking more risks than you should in servicing some of these clients.

You'll need to evaluate whether or not the weight of the weft and/or removing the bonded wefts will cause more damage to the client's own hair. Sometimes it is OK to sacrifice some of the client's own hair for the sake of the overall style. However, be sure of your client, and be sure of the service you'll be doing. If you suspect a client could be "abusive" – to their own hair, or might take legal action against you for further damage to their hair – do not do hair extension services for this client.

Oily Scalp – Oil Applied to Hair

People with an exceptionally oily scalp may not be able to wear adhesive bonded wefts. Some hair preparations that are oily can also cause the bond to break down and not adhere to the hair.

Also, the bond seems to break down faster on some individuals. The reason or reasons for this are not yet known. This problem cannot always be anticipated.

How to Know if It is Right

Because bonding can be so unpredictable, it can be helpful to you to do a test of the bond on your client before you do the complete style.

Put at least one strip of a weft in your client's hair. Have your client wear it for several days and through at least one shampooing. Testing the bonding method on your client before doing a complete style can save both you and your client a lot of time, money and disappointment.

Explain the Possible Problems to Your Client

Be sure to discuss these aspects of bonding with your client. Also, remember HAIR – H A I R – How Am I Responsible. Be a professional. Be sure of the products you use on your client's hair. Not all manufacturers or distributors of products used in the hair extension business disclose the ingredients in their products. Be careful: be professional.

ADVANTAGES AND DISADVANTAGES

Advantages

Probably one of the major advantages of the bonding technique is that it is quick and safe. In a short period of time, a client can have a head of thicker, fuller hair.

The bonding technique can be used to help a client decide if he or she should add highlights or lowlights to their hair. The bonding technique can be used for those weekly clients who need volume added to their hair in place of heavy teasing or back-brushing. Bonding can be used to create great "special occasion" styles – New Year's Eve, and so on.

Disadvantages

The major disadvantage to bonding is that it can be unpredictable. On some clients it just will not stay bonded to their hair. On other clients sometimes it will stay and other times it will come out with the first shampoo. I'm a perfect example of that. I've been able to wear wefts bonded in for as long as 6 weeks. Other times they just slide off the minute I have my hair shampooed. Since I don't change my hair care products, that's not the cause. However, I do take medications, and one guess I have is that could be the reason.

Stylists have told me that some of their customers seem to have problems with the bond staying in past 1-2 shampoos if the client is are under a great deal of stress.

Another disadvantage to bonding is relative to the recommended length of hair. The longer the hair, the more stress is placed on the client's own hair. The bonding technique is not recommended in this situation.

SUPPLIES

The following items are the supplies you will need to practice the bonding technique.

Manikin	Clips
Manikin holder	Hair dryer
Shears (used to cut weft)	Hair bond (adhesive)
Rattail comb	Weft of hair
Orangewood stick (optional)	Hair spray
Adhesive bond remover	

ATTACHING WEFTS

Preparation of Hair

The first step in all hair extension services is to prepare the weft. First, always shampoo the weft(s). Then proceed with any other services required, which may include conditioning, perming and/or coloring.

When doing clients, next, service your client's own hair, performing all necessary cleaning, conditioning and chemical services. It is recommended that you clean your client's hair with a deep cleansing shampoo to be sure that all residue and oils are removed.

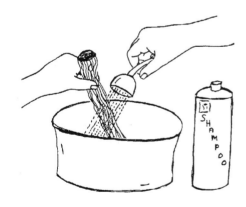

For practice on your Manikin, shampoo the hair and the weft. Be sure that both the hair and the weft are completely dry! Remember, bond will not stick to wet hair.

Sectioning Hair

The next step is to section the hair where you want to place the first weft. Clean partings are very important.

Be sure that you let the hair fall naturally.

On a Manikin, the hair direction is not that definite. However, when doing clients remember – don't bond against the growth pattern. If you do, the bonded wefts can cause stress to the roots of the client's hair. It also can be uncomfortable.

Remember, you build a style – starting at the bottom and moving up.

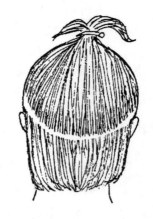

Measure Width of The Weft

Next measure the weft for the width of the track. When bonding, you will usually want to attach about 4" of weft (width) along the part at a time instead of a weft along the entire width of the track (part).

When doing client's hair there are several reasons for attaching smaller parts of a weft. These are: First, correct placement, (that is, closeness to part, yet on the hair) is easier and more accurate. Second, smaller sections reduce the amount of stress on the client's hair. Third, if only one side begins to slip, only one part of the track needs to be re-done.

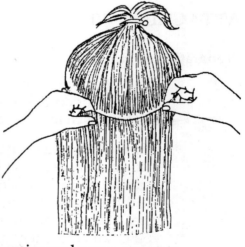

To measure the width of the weft, you hold the weft up to the hair, at the part.

Cut Weft

After measuring the exact amount of weft you'll need, cut it to fit.

Apply Bond To The Weft

DO NOT SHAKE the bottle of bond. Shaking it can change the molecular structure of the bond and cause it not to stick. Also, if the bond freezes or is subject to extreme temperatures, it will lose its adhesive properties.

Apply the bond at the top of the weft, on the stitching. It's difficult to explain how much adhesive to apply. However, it should be at least the width of the applicator. You need enough bond to insure that the bonding will hold, but not too much. (This causes problems with bond seeping onto the scalp or onto hair not part of the tracking area. Also too much bond creates problems when trying to remove the bonding.)

Mark the Spots

To mark the area where you will be placing bond on the hair, hold the weft up, bonded side toward the hair and lightly touch the ends to the hair. This then "marks" the spots at either end of where you will apply bond to the hair. Put the weft back down and go to the next step.

Apply Bond To the Hair

Next, apply bond to the hair, on the hair next to the scalp, just below the parting. If you accidentally get any bond on loose hair, be sure to remove it by wiping it off with your fingers.

Practice being neat. When doing clients, loose hairs caught in the bonded track will be uncomfortable and will eventually cause these hairs to pull loose from your client's scalp.

Apply Bond Again To Weft

Then, apply bond again to the weft. The first application of bond will have soaked into the weft. This light second coat insures better bonding of the weft to the hair. Beware that you do not put too much bond on the weft.

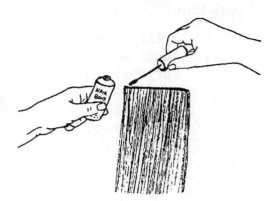

Place Weft On the Hair

Place the bonded side of the weft on top of the bond on the hair.

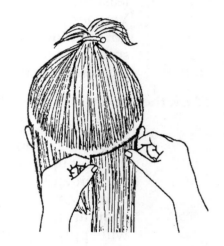

Securing the Weft

You can use the end of your rat-tail comb or an orangewood stick to press it down firmly in place. Also, after you have completed the track, with a blow dryer, dry the area for a few minutes.

Repeat for Each Track

For the complete style, repeat the attachment of each weft, starting from the bottom and building up. Remember you need to have enough hair to cover the wefts.

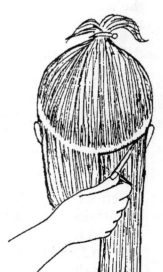

Setting/Fixing the Bond

After all wefts have been attached, place your Manikin (your client) under a hair dryer for about 15 minutes to make sure that the bond is completely dry.

Cut and Style

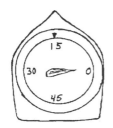

After the bond has had a chance to set, you will then proceed to cut and style your new creation.
(See Chapter 7 regarding cutting and styling techniques.)

MAINTAINING AND RE-DOING THE STYLE

Remove with Adhesive Bond Remover

Apply Remover to Top of Weft
Remember, bonding on each client will be different. Each time you remove wefts, even on the same client, it may be different. Sometimes the wefts come off easily, other times with more difficulty. Your objective is to loosen the bond enough to slide the wefts off.

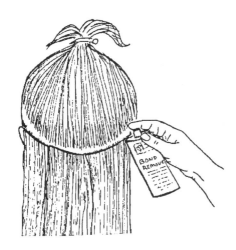

Use an adhesive bond remover. This kind of remover contains mineral oil. You can also use hair spray or wig luster spray that contains mineral oil. First spray the top of the weft, at the area bonded.

Apply Remover Under Weft
Next, lift the weft up and spray the area that is bonded from underneath. Leave the spray on the hair and weft from 5 to 10 minutes before attempting to remove the weft.

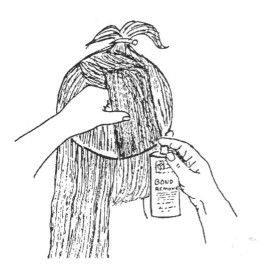

Work Weft Away from Scalp

Gently work the weft away from the hair. You will want to SLIDE the weft down the hair shaft. If the weft resists, re-apply the adhesive bond remover.

Other Removal Option

If the weft will not release using the adhesive bond remover or you don't have any available, there are two alternative removal methods to use. One technique is to apply a mixture of shampoo and conditioner to the bonded area. The second (and least preferred) technique is to apply mineral oil (or baby oil) to the bonded area. First, shampoo the entire head.

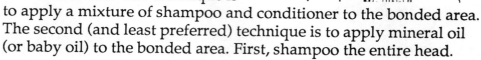

Apply to Top of Weft
Then apply the shampoo-conditioner mixture with your working fingers to the bonded area on top. If you must use oil, you may need to use cotton or an eye dropper to apply the oil, then rub it into the top area.

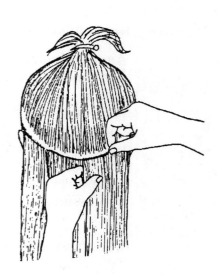

Apply to Underside of Weft
Next, apply either the shampoo-conditioner mixture or the oil to the underside of the weft at the point where the weft is bonded.

Slide the Weft Off
Gently pull down – never tug or use a lot of pressure – on the weft to slide it off the client's hair.

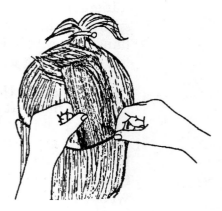

Removing Residue

No matter what technique you use, there may be a residue of bond on the hair. Use a fine-tooth comb to remove it.

On the wefts, pick-off the residue of the bond. You don't have to worry about removing all of the old bond. However, if you have had to use oil to remove the wefts, you will want to make sure that you remove all the oil and any of the bond that has "jelled" and contains some of the oil. This may be difficult, requiring the use of a detergent and a toothbrush. Apply the detergent to the bond, and with the toothbrush, brush away from the hair on the weft.

Or, you can always purchase new hair.

Service Weft and Reapply

If you are going to reuse the wefts, be sure to deep-condition them, and, if needed, enhance the color, then dry. After your client's hair is cleaned, conditioned and any other services are done, be sure the client's hair is also completely dry.

Reapply the wefts to the hair. Remember to place them in a slightly different location from where they were previously placed.

GENERAL COMMENTS

Test Strip

Remember, you can save yourself and your client a lot of grief if you do a test strip on your client. First, you need to know if bond will adhere to your client's own hair. Second, you need to determine if your client has any sensitivity to bond.

Hair Captured in Bond

Right at the beginning (during your consultation), explain to your client that everyone loses hair naturally every day. As a result, since the bond is on the hair, hairs that would have been shed naturally will be captured in the adhesive bond.

Weft Drag

Beware of "weft drag." This happens when the weft begins to slip or grows out. If the weft is more than 1" to 1 1/2" away from the scalp, the weft is putting too much stress on the roots of the hair and can pull hair out. Be sure to have your client return in one week for a free check-up appointment. They must also return in at least 6 weeks to see how much drag the weft may be causing. You may make this part of your agreement with your client.

Understand Bonding

Bonding can be an excellent technique to use for many of your clients. Like all things in life – it has its good points and its drawbacks. It can be unpredictable at times. But, with experience, you'll be able to better understand which clients and what hairstyles are most appropriate for the bonding technique.

I personally believe that there will be a great deal of "bread-and-butter" business doing bonding on women or men over 35 years of age. This group has generally lost some of their hair and wants thicker hair – more volume. Also, these women and men often lead busy lives and don't have time to daily set and style their hair. Hair added for volume can insure that their style will last for a week – reducing the time they have to spend caring for their own hair. It's definitely worth the money to the busy woman or man!

SUMMARY

The bonding technique is not appropriate for all clients because of sensitivity to latex, oily scalp or weak or overly damaged hair.

It is suggested that you do a test strip on a client before doing a complete style. Insist that clients return regularly so that the wefts can be checked to prevent undue stress to the client's hair.

Chapter 5

PERMING FOR HAIR EXTENSIONS

INTRODUCTION

Better Than ...

As I address this chapter, the first thing that comes to my mind is that stylists doing hair extension services must be "better than the average bear – ho, ho, ho." Perming? Sure, everyone knows how to perm. Well, the truth is that when you get into hair extension services – you have to know more than you realize.

Remember, you really are going to *create magic!* Now, when your client asks for it – you can create a miracle, an unbelievable transformation.

All the successful stylists I know doing hair extension services tell me that they really like their clients. Their hair extension clients are appreciative, listen to them and are not only willing – but extremely interested in reaching out for a newer, more exciting look.

An Advanced Specialty

As a person doing hair extension services, you are really a specialist – an advanced specialist. Beyond knowing various attachment techniques and understanding their appropriate uses – you are a chemical services specialist and a cutting/styling specialist. You must be an expert in all the disciplines within our industry.

A hair extension specialist's business is based on a very human, natural desire to *want what we don't have*. Clients who have extremely curly hair usually want less curl. Clients who have straight hair usually want curl. People with thick, long hair sometimes want even more hair. But think of all those people who have thin, fine hair. People who can't grow it want long hair. You can give it to them. Our entire business is based on giving people what they don't have.

As someone who specializes in hair extension services you must become an expert in dealing with the curl in your client's hair – and in the hair to be added. Actually, many times you can reduce the number of chemical treatments on your client's hair by accomplishing the desired results with hair extensions.

SUPPLIES

The following are the supplies you will need to perm wefts.

Manikin and holder	Perm solution and neutralizer
Plastic bag	Timer
Wide-tooth comb	Rubber gloves
Rattail comb	T-pins
Clips	Perm manufacturer's products chart
End papers	Pre-cleansing shampoo
Perm rods	Human hair weft

FACTS TO KNOW ABOUT WEFTS

You Maintain Control

There are two ways to deal with the quality of hair you are going to use on a client. These are:

1. Purchase the hair yourself.
2. Have your client purchase the hair.

If you have your client purchase the hair, and you provide only attachment and styling services, I believe that you have limited yourself to a less professional status than you deserve. Hair that is brought to you by a client places a considerable degree of risk on you. You cannot take the risks involved in doing chemical services to this unknown product. You cannot be assured of the performance of this product. You cannot even be sure whether the product is 100% human hair or blended with synthetics. Do you allow your clients to provide their own chemical products? Do you not make a margin of profit on the professional products you use on your client's hair?

I believe that if you are a specialist, you take responsibility for all aspects of your service. This includes the hair that you are going to add. So, if you purchase the hair yourself, you know the properties of the hair. You know what you can and cannot do to the hair. You are in control!

Most Hair Used Will Need to Be Permed

The curl in the hair that you use in your hair extension services is often a very important consideration relative to the finished style.

You can buy hair that is straight or pre-curled. Most hair used in hair extensions is either Chinese or Indian. Both of these are a brownish-black color (not jet-black). Chinese hair is very straight. Indian hair has a natural wave. If the style you want to achieve features straight hair then you can use Chinese hair without a perm. If the style you want will have a slight wave then you can use Indian hair. Otherwise the hair will need to be permed.

Factory Permed Versus Custom Perming

If you can purchase hair that has the curl you need for the style you are planning, you can save yourself the time required to perm the wefts.

On the other hand, if you want a unique type of curl, then you are better off customizing the hair for your client's needs by perming the weft yourself. In fact, you can match any texture of hair to your client's own hair. Or, you can create the texture that the client wants, which may not be possible with their own hair. This may be the reason your client wants hair extensions. Perming the hair for your client's hair extensions gives you, the stylist, ultimate control of the total finished style.

Hair That Cannot/Should Not Be Permed

Not all wefts are 100% human hair, as they are represented. If there is any synthetic fiber blended into the weft, it will not perm properly.

Also, you cannot perm all hair that is available because some of it has been colored. The method used to color this hair is called chrome dyeing. Hair that has been chrome dyed can be difficult to perm.

First, the hair shaft may be so coated that the permanent wave solution may not penetrate correctly or evenly.

In addition, when trying to perm hair that has been dyed, there is a very good chance that the hair will turn green.

Just like with client's hair – it is hazardous to try to perm hair that is in a weakened or dry condition. Since most of the hair you'll be using was brownish-black to start with, any other colors are a result of decolorizing (bleaching) of the hair. Imagine if you decolorized a client's hair ten levels – from black to light blonde. What condition would you expect that hair to be in? That's not saying you can't perm light blonde hair – you just have to be very knowledgeable, skilled and careful. Always do a test strand first!

Unique Features of the Hair You Purchase

Yes, the hair in a 100% human hair weft that is not colored with a chrome dye is just like your client's hair and can be treated as such – with the following unique characteristics:

Porosity of Cuticle

Most of the hair you will buy has been processed with part of the cuticle removed. (See Chapter 1.) Since all perming solutions must pass through the cuticle before they work on the cortex, special consideration should be given to the porosity of the cuticle. In most cases, hair in the wefts can be considered to have high porosity of the cuticle. After doing your pre-perm analysis of the weft, you may want to treat excessive porosity by applying fillers before perming.

Porosity of Cortex

The reason the cuticle has been reduced is to prevent matting. If the hair were what is called root-turned or cut-hair, then the cuticle on the hair would be going the same direction, but in wefts it is not. The root-ends and the hair-ends are all mixed up. You have no way of knowing which ends are up. The porosity of the cortex is often affected by the age of the hair and longer hair is older. In older hair there may be air spaces present in the cortex.

When perm solution enters these spaces, the solution will process too rapidly. In addition it can cause a rapid breakdown of the keratin, since there are fewer S-bonds in these spaces.

A technique used to even out the porosity is to allow for what is referred to later in this chapter as the 15 minute molecular flow period.

First you thoroughly rinse the hair with warm water for 15 minutes.

Next you towel-blot the hair.

Then, you wait 15 minutes before applying the neutralizer. The reason for this is that the porous part of the cortex holds more water which will dilute the permanent wave solution.

PRE-PERM ANALYSIS

The First Step

Before doing hair extension services, you will do a consultation with your client (Chapter 8). Part of your consultation will be a pre-perm analysis. This is required for your client's own hair. Then, after you purchase the hair you will be adding, you also have to go through the same steps of a pre-perm analysis for this hair.

A pre-perm analysis allows you to do a diagnosis of exactly what you can (and cannot) do to achieve the look you and your client desire. It involves an evaluation of the hair's condition relative to porosity, elasticity, texture, density, body and length.

Checking Porosity

Porosity can be checked very simply by holding the hair between the thumb and forefinger of one hand and gently sliding the thumb and forefinger of the other hand down the hair shaft. If it feels rather slick you know that it's probably resistant. If you get a little bit of ruffling, you'll know that there is some porosity there. The greater the degree of ruffling, the greater the degree of porosity. Porosity affects the speed with which a perm will process.

Usually you will consider the hair on a weft to be medium to highly porous hair.

Checking Elasticity

The second thing you have to consider is the elasticity of the hair. To determine the elasticity you hold the end of a hair between your thumb and forefinger and slightly pull it. If it breaks rather easily, it probably has no elasticity. Hair with good elasticity will take a good perm. Hair with poor elasticity will take only a moderately good perm. If it has no elasticity (the hair breaks rather easily), it should not be permed.

Be particularly critical of the elasticity of hair wefts in the light shades. Once permanent wave solution is applied, the hair begins to soften. This hair can easily be overstretched by tight winding or pulling. Hair that is overstretched will not return to its former length and will be damaged and weakened.

Checking Texture

Texture refers to the feel of the hair and includes a number of distinct properties. However, usually when evaluating texture in preparation for a perm, the diameter of each individual hair is the main consideration. It can be fine, medium fine, medium, medium coarse or coarse.

Checking Density

Density, hair per square inch on the head, is an important factor in the wrapping/blocking of the perm. On a weft, the density can be related to the thickness of the weft. You can control the density somewhat by limiting the amount of hair you perm at one time. In general, you could consider a weft fairly dense.

Checking Body

The amount of body is the next thing to consider. You'll be evaluating your client's hair for old perms and how much out-growth there is. You'll also check how much natural wave there is, etc.

On a weft, it is easy to observe how straight Chinese hair is and to see the natural wave in Indian hair.

Length to be Considered

As far as length goes, when perming a weft, any hair that is 6" or longer is considered long hair and the type of wrap required for long hair is different from that for short hair. Long hair presents more problems in the following areas; maintaining tension when wrapping, correct saturation of the perm solution and correct rinsing.

SELECTING THE PERM PRODUCT

Categories of Perms

Throughout the industry there are basically three categories of perms. They are:

Conventional alkaline perm
Buffered conventional perm
Acid perm

Alkaline perms in the conventional and buffered conventional categories use ammonium-thioglycolate as the main active ingredient. This gives a crisper curl and is a stronger product than the acid perm.

Acid perms generally give a softer result and treat the hair more gently. There is a direct relationship between the porosity of the hair, the lotion (perm) selected and the processing time. The main active ingredient is ammonium glycerol monothioglycolate – referred to as GMT.

Using the Results of Your Analysis

The porosity, elasticity and texture are all considerations in picking the proper perm. The appropriate product for particular hair types is the key to the success of the whole design.

It is important to remember that there is a direct relationship between the porosity of the hair, the length of time that the perm solution is to be left on and the strength of the solution that you select.

Understanding the Hair in Wefts

Applying the information about wefts you now have, as well as information about perm products, there are some generalizations that can be made about which are the correct products to use on wefts.

First, dark colors can be permed with either alkaline or acid products. Second, you will want to consider an acid perm (which is milder) for longer hair (which is older).

Evaluating the Features of Perms

In selecting the correct product, you need to be aware of all the various features of several manufacturers' product lines. Probably one of the more difficult things a stylist (like all consumers today) must do is to cut through the sales hype.

Unfortunately, we must dig through a battery of adjectives that tell us about the "sizzle" of the product without providing the necessary chemical information. The following are some of the basic considerations you will want to apply when selecting a product.

Strength of Product Exactly what pH level is required to accomplish your objective or to accommodate the needs and the condition of the hair you are perming? An alkaline product has a higher pH level, whereas an acid perm product has a lower pH level.

Pre-Wrap Feature Some products are designed to help equalize the porosity of the hair by providing a pre-wrap lotion. If this feature is not part of the product and you feel it is needed, is there a suggested pre-conditioning regime that would be appropriate?

Temperature Requirements It is helpful to know how a product will work with and without the addition of heat. Sometimes you may have to consider the environment (temperature and humidity) where you are working and make adjustments accordingly. (Usually when perming wefts, you do not use heat.)

WRAPPING TECHNIQUES

Basic Considerations

If you wind the hair too tightly on the rod, you can overstretch the hair during processing. This can damage the hair.

Since the curl will tend to follow the diameter of the rods, selection of the rods should be made carefully.

Suggestions

Although you may use any of several wrapping techniques; oval (croquignole wrap), piggyback wrap and others. Most stylists perming wefts have found that the spiral wrapping technique is the best.

The most successful perming I've seen has been done on two types of rods. The first is the straight rod – wrapped using the spiral technique, distributing the hair back and forth on the rod.

The second technique which is very popular and very successful, involves using a long rod – wrapping the hair in a way that none of the hair overlaps. This assures complete and consistent perm lotion saturation.

HOW TO PERM WEFTS

Perming Wefts on Client's Head

Do not perm the wefts on the client's head. If you have attached the wefts on a braided track, there is too great a risk of getting perm solution into the braided hair, which could damage the client's hair. If the wefts are bonded in, the perm solution can affect the adhesive properties the bond and you also run the risk of trapping perm lotion under the top of the weft. If you have used the individual braiding technique, you are again dealing with the possibility of seriously damaging the client's own hair that is captured in the braid, etc.

Prepare the Weft

Always shampoo the weft when you receive it. Because it has traveled many thousands of miles, chances are the hair is very dusty.

If you feel the hair needs conditioning, which usually is the case, be sure to do so, using restructuring rather than a moisturizing conditioner.

Be gentle when shampooing a weft. Do not rub the hair. It is easier to handle if you keep the weft together in a bundle.

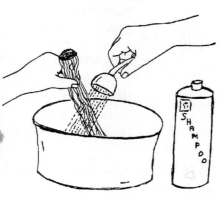

Use a Manikin Head to Hold Weft

Most Manikins manufactured today have a polyurethane filled head. This type of construction allows you to use your Manikin for not only braiding and styling practice, but also as a head to which you can affix your weft.

To protect the hair on the Manikin's head from the perm lotion, cover it with a plastic bag. A small trash bag will work very well.

Fold the Weft

The width of the weft you are working with may be as much as 108". If the width of the weft is greater than the circumference of the Manikin's head, fold the weft in half, joining the two ends together.

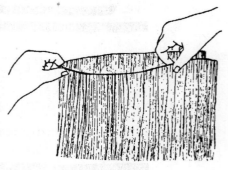

T-pin the Weft to the Manikin Head

Starting above the ear, attach the weft to the head by inserting T-pins into the sewing on the top of the weft. Space the T-pins 2" to 3" apart. If the width of the weft (even folded in half) is greater than the circumference of the head, when you reach the point where you began, T-pin the remaining weft just above the previous row.

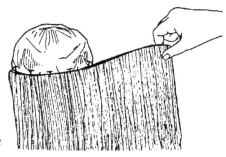

Do a Test Strand

Remember, every weft is different. After you have done your pre-perm analysis and select the perm you think is best – do a test strand.

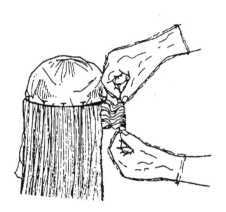

Wrap the Perm

Follow all the basic principles of wrapping a perm. Be aware of the tension, stress points, positioning, correct distribution of the hair on the rod, etc. If you have pinned the weft around the head more than one time, treat each layer separately. One of the things most stylists forget is that usually one weft contains as much hair as is on a client's head – only it's concentrated on one weft. Keep this in mind when sectioning the hair and take small enough sections so you can get proper penetration.

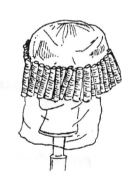

You can come close to matching any hair texture. Obviously, it's difficult to match it exactly. In many cases, you will be altering the degree of curl in both the client's hair and the weft. The most important consideration in matching texture, is the rod selection, because it's the rod size that gives you the curl size.

There are many kinds of rods: benders, spiral rods, zig-zag rods, crimping rods, and so on. New products are always fun to try.

It's interesting and exciting to see what new things you can do with hair. However, new products/tools should all be tested before you actually use them on your client. Trying them on a weft is an excellent way to see how they work.

The best wrapping technique is a spiral wrap.

Apply Perm Solution

If your strand test is satisfactory, apply the lotion to all the curls. Be sure to read the manufacturer's instructions. One of the reasons for most perm problems is that stylists get in a rush and don't take the time to read the directions.

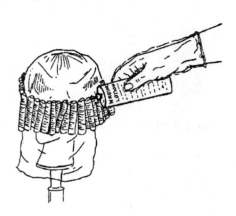

A helpful hint – push a T-pin into the top of your applicator bottle instead of using a scissors to cut it. This gives you a smaller hole in the top, which helps you to regulate the flow.

Cover with Plastic Bag

In all cases, cover the rods with a plastic bag. Even if the manufacturer's instructions call for placing the client's head under a dryer – for perming wefts **DO NOT put under a dryer.** Instead, cover the rods with a plastic bag.

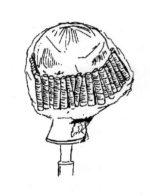

Take Test Curls

Do test curls **EVERY 2 MINUTES.** The wefts are Chinese or Indian hair, remember, the hair has been processed and has had part of its cuticle removed. If it's not brownish-black it has been decolorized (bleached). Because of this you must watch the processing very closely. Never leave the weft – stay with it through the processing period. Chinese hair has a tendency to process quickly.

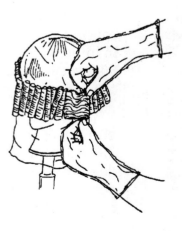

When Processing Is Completed

After the desired curl has been achieved, before you rinse – set your timer for 15 minutes.

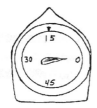

Thoroughly Rinse the Hair

Thoroughly rinse the hair. (Don't soak it – rinse it.) Rinsing is extremely important for 3 reasons:

1. starts the bonding process
2. promotes better curl formation
3. alleviates post-perm odor

Although most instructions read "rinse for 5 minutes" – you MUST rinse for **15 minutes.** Incomplete rinsing and not enough blotting are probably the major causes of improper perming and damaged hair.

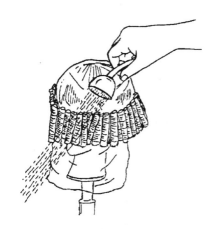

Thoroughly Blot

With a towel, thoroughly blot the hair. You do not want to dry the hair, but you do want to remove all excess water.

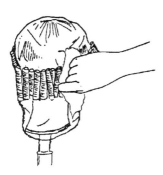

Fifteen-Minute Wait

This 15 minute waiting period is what is called the molecular flow period. This time allows for the maximum number of bonds to slip by and come back into a closer proximity, so when the perm is completely neutralized, the hair will be supported with as many bonds reformed as possible. Also, this time helps deal with problems with the porosity of the hair cortex.

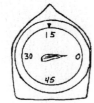

Blot Again

After the 15 minute molecular flow period, blot again.

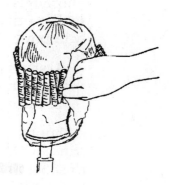

Neutralizing

When you apply the neutralizer, you start on the bottom row. It's very important to thoroughly saturate each and every curl. You go over and under each rod as you work, being careful not to miss any rods. You'll leave the neutralizer on according to manufacturer's instructions – usually 5 minutes.

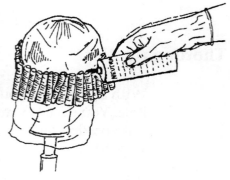

Rinse with Rods

Then, with the rods still in place, rinse for 5 minutes. The reason you do not remove the rods when rinsing is that it is easier.

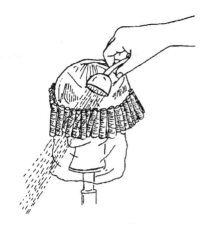

Rinse without Rods

Next, remove the rods and and rinse for 1 minute more. Do not shampoo.

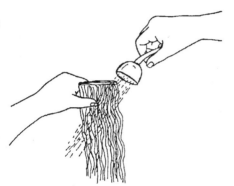

I can't emphasize enough that you really need to rinse the hair. I have seen countless problems as a result of improper rinsing.

Note: if possible, wait 24-48 hours before coloring or attaching to the client's hair.

BECOMING AN EXPERT

When Did You Last ...?

When did you last study anything about perming? Probably when you were in school. And, this was probably not your favorite class – so many things to learn! You were probably more anxious to get to styling – the fun part.

If you are going to be a hair extension expert you'll need to be a curl expert. You'll need to understand how to achieve all types of curl patterns in your client's own hair and in the hair for the extensions.

Back to Basics

When it comes to hair chemistry – chances are you'll need to return briefly to basics – back to the things you've forgotten – before you can advance to becoming an expert. There are a number of publications available that can be extremely helpful. I'd recommend Milady's publications:

Hair Structure and Chemistry Simplified
Milady's Black Cosmetology

Manufacturers as a Resource

One excellent source for advanced education is manufacturers. Many companies have expert instructors out in the field who will come to your salon or school and give you specific classes. You can learn everything from basics to complete product-line information.

I particularly like classes with stylists who are actively working at a salon but who also do teaching work for manufacturers as a part-time job.

You're Not Alone

Many, I mean many, stylists I've talked to say they just don't want to perm the wefts. They want ready-permed hair to use. It's not the money (usually you can charge extra for this service). Sometimes it's the limited space available to stylists in the salon where they work. I always feel so sorry for stylists who only have the top of the washing machine or dryer on which to work. Sometimes it's the time – they haven't allotted enough time in their book for additional services to the hair. Sometimes it's availability of product. A lot of salons, particularly those with a rental station arrangement, just don't have enough of a product line readily available to the stylists.

But, the basic, the underlying, the real reason that most stylists opt for pre-permed hair is simply that they don't have enough confidence in the product they are going to perm and in their perming capabilities. If both these negatives are corrected – if the stylist can find a source of hair that is permable – and if the stylist can become an expert in perming – this stylist can really be in control – can be an expert par excellence in hair extension services.

SUMMARY

Hair has many features, color, texture, density, porosity and so on. But, hair has no sex. And, hair has no race. No matter who needs more hair, you can help them.

Remember, every weft has its own personality. Do a pre-perm analysis and always do a test strand. Be sure to select the correct perm for the curl you want and for the color of the weft you are perming. It is important to wrap the perm with consistent tension. T-pin the weft to a Manikin head, then wrap. Never leave the weft. Be sure to stay with it during the complete processing time. More wefts are destroyed because the stylist didn't keep checking the curl. Rinse and rinse and rinse. Another major mistake that is made when perming wefts is that the weft is not rinsed enough!

Go back to basics and become an expert in perming. It will help tremendously in all aspects of your business and it is very important relative to hair extension services!

Chapter 6

COLORING FOR HAIR EXTENSIONS

INTRODUCTION

Seven Out of Ten Women and Men ...

Now, color is an important part of our daily living. It's all around us. It's estimated that at least seven out of every ten women and men color their hair at least once in their lifetime.

The public has accepted that coloring hair is as much a part of hair care as shampooing. Since I was raised with many aunts who were hairstylists, I thought professional hair care was a normal way of life. I also grew up not knowing there was any stigma attached to coloring hair. My mother wanted redheaded children and none of her six children were born with red hair. I was ten years old before I discovered that not everyone used a "special" red-colored rinse after shampooing.

It was an absolute surprise when I went into the business myself in the early 1960s and discovered that perming and coloring hair was sometimes "something that you just don't do unless ..."

Coloring Still Needs Expanding and Promotion

Recently, I was reviewing some teaching materials prepared by the salon educational director of one of the large department store chains. The entire program, an excellent presentation, is geared to help their stylists learn how to sell and use color in their salons. Here was something I assumed, at least by now, was just a natural. Doesn't every stylist sell and promote hair coloring? Another awakening.

By the way, within a few months of launching this educational program, the chain salon started seeing a *15% increase in sales* in coloring services.

Back To Basics

To be truly successful in the rapidly growing hair extension business – you really do have to go back to basics! Dull, you think? No way! The basics are the foundation of everything.

Coloring in hair extension services usually means working with both the client's hair and the hair extensions. Although coloring for this service is

Coloring in hair extension services usually means working with both the client's hair and the hair extensions. Although coloring for this service is similar to coloring on a client's own hair – there are some very important differences and factors which you will learn about in this chapter.

SUPPLIES

Play-Doh®
Color products
Rubber gloves
Small mixing bowls
Large mixing bowls
Wide-tooth comb
Rattail comb

Applicator brush
Measuring cup or bottle
Plastic wrap
Plastic bag
Manikin or head
Manikin holder
T-pins

Note: Play-Doh® is manufactured by Kenner Parker Toys and is available at most toy and hobby stores. We have tried other brands of modeling compounds but find that they are not true to color for doing the exercises shown on Figures 1, 2 and 3 in this chapter.

FACTS TO KNOW ABOUT WEFTS

The Original Hair Color

The starting point is to understand the original hair color of the wefts, the hair you will be adding. Since a majority of the hair used is either Chinese or Indian, and since these types of hair are originally a brownish-black – that means all other colors available are colors created first by decolorizing (bleaching) the hair.

Stages of Lightening

Of course, not all the confusion about coloring is due to a lack of information. Some of the problems have to do with inconsistent or conflicting terminology. There is a very strong movement to standardize terms. But I'm afraid it will be several years before this is accomplished.

You can talk with manufacturers, educators, instructors, writers in the field, and you will get different answers to the questions of –

Stages of Lightening (decolorization, bleaching)
Levels of Color
Shades of Color

As an example, several textbooks discuss the seven stages of lightening with stage 1 being black. Other charts show ten stages of lightening, with stage 1 (the first stage of lightening) a dark brown. Well, when describing the stages of lightening of the Chinese or Indian hair I find I have to use the chart that shows ten stages to be able to sufficiently describe the various stages the black hair goes through as it is decolorized.

COLORING FOR HAIR EXTENSIONS

The hair's natural color is brownish-black (not a jet-black). It contains molecules from all the primary colors – *blue, red* and *yellow*.

The first stage of lightening (stage 1) is a dark brown, some of the blue molecules have been lifted.

Stage 2 is a result of the bleach lifting out more blue molecules and the hair becomes a reddish brown.

At stage 3 the hair lightens to a brownish red (more red than brown).

Through stages 4, 5, 6 and 7 more and more of the red molecules are removed by the bleach.

At stage 8 the hair is now yellow orange – just a few of the red molecules are left.

Then, at stage 9 (yellow) almost all the red molecules have been lifted.

Stage 10 is described as pale yellow. Even some of the yellow molecules have been lifted at this stage. However, the Chinese or Indian hair can become over processed by this point – it is weak and may not survive any additional chemical services. It may also be dry and may break.

Factory Colored versus Custom Coloring

Much of the hair that is sold for hair extensions is pre-colored at a factory – either the source that is involved in selling the hair or the factory that will sew the weft. Some factories do both.

At the factory, hair is colored by dying it with a chrome dye. These metallic dyes are not professional colors. The reason metallic dye is used is to prevent or reduce fading of the color. The factory will do 10 to 20 different dye lots. Then these colors are blended together to create the final colors that are sold.

However, there is also hair available that has not been dyed but has only been lightened. This hair is designed to be custom colored by the stylist to match the client's own hair color.

Advantages of Factory Dyed Hair

There is only one advantage to hair that is dyed at the factory. It saves time for the stylist. There are usually from 15 to 35 final colors created by blending the basic dyed colors.

Disadvantages of Factory Dyed Hair

The disadvantage of hair that is dyed is that it cannot safely be re-colored or even highlighted or lowlighted.

You can test hair to see if it has been chrome dyed. Cut a strand of it. Immerse it in a solution of 20 volume peroxide and 20 drops of ammonia for 30 minutes. Remove the hair, dry it and observe the strand. Sometimes hair that is dyed either will not change color or will lighten in spots.

The length of time necessary for penetration may damage the hair and coloring (or perming) it generally means an uneven and/or unpredictable result.

Advantages of Custom Coloring

The advantages of the stylist custom coloring the hair to be used in extension services are obvious. The stylist has complete control – can match perfectly the client's hair and/or create the real color the client wants which may be an entirely different color. The stylist has no restrictions and can highlight or lowlight, decolorize or tint or tone the hair so it will be natural and undetectable from the client's own hair.

Disadvantages of Stylist Coloring

There really are none, if you understand coloring. It's easy when you have all the information and you practice.

Hair That Cannot/Should Not Be Colored

Hair that has been factory dyed cannot be "counted on". That is, you don't know what you are dealing with. Is this hair that has been decolorized (bleached) all the way out – then colored darker? Is this hair that has been blended with other dyed hair? There is no way to guarantee you can cover up the chrome dyes used. There is also no way to guarantee you can remove these dyes. In days gone by, to color wigs, we used dye designed to dye fabrics. Of course, the results were that we acheived various shades of black and dark brown without much luster. This is because in the '60s most, if not all, wigs were made with chrome dyed hair.

Besides not knowing exactly what the hair is like "under" the dye. Metallic dyes (used for factory dyed hair) penetrate the cortex and combine with the sulphur bonds. As a result, the sulphur bonds are no longer available for permanent waving. Also, metallic salts react violently with hydrogen peroxide.

If there is any synthetic fiber blended into the hair, you cannot color this hair. You can only color 100% human hair.

Other hair that you may not be able to successfully color is hair that has been overprocessed at the factory.

Unique Features of the Hair You Purchase

Again, the hair on a 100% human hair weft that is not colored with a chrome dye is similar to your client's hair and can be treated as such. As discussed earlier in this book, part of the cuticle has been removed, so this hair can be considered to have high porosity of the cuticle.

If the color of the hair is anything other than a brownish-black, then you know the hair has been decolorized (bleached). This means you will usually be working in what is called a tint-back environment. Some of the color molecules have been removed from the hair. To achieve the colors you want, you may have to replace the missing color molecules.

PRE-COLOR ANALYSIS

In addition to your basic questions/preparations relative to your client's own hair coloring needs ie: condition of scalp, patch test – there are five questions to ask yourself when conducting your pre-color analysis for both the client's hair and the hair for their extensions. These are:

1. What is the natural shade of the hair?
2. What is the percentage of gray?
3. What is the porosity?
4. What is the texture of the hair?
5. What is the desired shade?

ABOUT COLOR PRODUCTS

Introduction

Every hair color can be categorized and organized into ten natural shade levels, from black on up to palest blonde. Hair color products are also organized according to the ten natural shade levels and according to six base colors, which are the primary and the secondary colors.

There are four classifications of color products. These are:

1. Temporary
2. Semi-permanent
3. Permanent
4. Progressive dyes

Temporary rinses put color on the hair shaft. They wash out with shampooing. They are a way of "sparking up" or adding depth to a color on the client's own hair and/or the hair extensions. Consider temporary rinses for that special occasion hairstyle.

Semi-permanent colors coat the hair shaft and deposit a little color which will fade with shampooing. However, semi-permanent products are excellent to use on hair for hair extensions. The reasons for this are, first, this coloring technique is gentle to the hair, which is important. Second, because of the porosity of processed Chinese and/or Indian hair, semi-permanent hair colors really do an excellent job of depositing color and the color lasts a lot longer than color usually does on client's hair.

Permanent color lasts longer, but will fade in time. Again, because of the porosity of the hair for hair extensions, fading (if properly colored) is not a serious problem. However, most of the time, your objective is to deposit color, not to lighten, so consider using lower volume peroxides, or dilute the peroxide with water.

Progressive dyes are not considered a professional product and are definitely not recommended for hair extensions.

THE RULES

Do You Remember?

Something you learned in school. Do you remember it? Chances are it's one of those things you use daily but can't explain to someone else. Just like the law of gravity (what goes up must come down) – the law of color never changes – but it cannot be explained quite as simply.

The Law of Color

Opposite each primary color is a secondary color which contains the other two primary colors. To neutralize any color, simply add the missing primary color or colors.

Do The Law of Color Exercise

On the next page is a work sheet. Use Play-Doh® in the three primary colors. Here is how you do it.

1. Make a small (1/2") ball of each of the primary colors – red, yellow and blue.

2. Place a small piece of yellow on the "Y" circle; red on the "R" circle and blue on the "B" circle. (Figure 1)

3. Mix equal parts yellow and red to get orange.

4. Divide the orange in half. Place one of the half pieces of orange on the "O" circle (Figure 2) and save the remaining half of orange for later.

5. Mix equal parts of red and blue to create violet.

6. Divide the violet in half. Place one of the half pieces of violet on the "V" circle (Figure 2) and save the remaining half of violet for later.

7. Mix equal parts of blue and yellow to get green.

8. Divide the green in half. Place one of the half pieces of green on the "G" circle (Figure 2) and save the remaining half of green for later.

9. Reread "The Law of Color" above – then do it.

10. Mix a piece of red and green. Roll the mixture in your hands and make a small strip. These colors will cancel or neutralize each other, creating a flesh colored beige. Place the strip on the dotted line between the "G" and "R" circles (Figure 3).

11. Take a piece of blue and orange. Roll and mix until a neutral color is achieved. Make into a small strip and place on the dotted line between the "B" and "O" circles (Figure 3).

12. Mix a piece of yellow and violet. Place the strip on the dotted line between the "Y" and "V" circles (Figure 3).

COLORING FOR HAIR EXTENSIONS

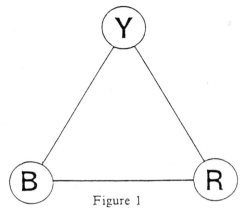

Figure 1

Primary Colors
The colors used to make all other colors.
RED – YELLOW – BLUE

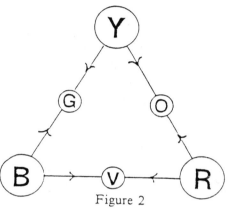

Figure 2

Secondary Colors
Mixtures of two primary colors.
GREEN = BLUE & YELLOW
VIOLET = BLUE & RED
ORANGE = RED & YELLOW

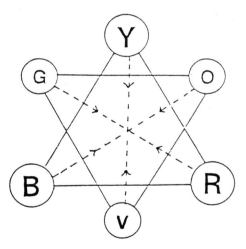

Figure 3

RED neutralizes GREEN
VIOLET neutralizes YELLOW
BLUE neutralizes ORANGE
GREEN neutralizes RED
YELLOW neutralizes VIOLET
ORANGE neutralizes BLUE

Applying The Law of Color

You will have to constantly remember this law of color to evaluate first, what color the weft is now – what has been removed from the previously brownish-black hair – and what do you need to add to the hair to get the desired results?

HOW TO COLOR WEFTS

Depending on the level of color you are trying to acheive, you may need to pre-lighten the weft before applying color to the hair. Just like on your client's hair, you will make the decision as to how much color may need to be lifted. Can you lift to the level and shade desired? Will you need to also deposit color? How much color?

Remember that when tints are combined with a developer (peroxide), an oxidation process begins. There is a lifting of the melanin that is the natural hair pigment, and there is a deposit of new color.

There are some "tricks" that can help you with coloring hair wefts for hair extensions.

What Color to Start With?

It helps to purchase factory lightened (bleached) wefts. Of course, you can take a brownish-black weft and decolorize (lighten) it yourself. However, the threads on the top of the weft will not change color to match the weft.

When selecting a weft color, choose a pre-lightened color that is closest to the final color you want.

Perm First, Color Second

Just as with your client's hair – remember, perm first and color second. If you are going to perm and then lighten the weft, be sure to use a smaller size rod for your perm because you'll lose some of the curl. Also, wait 24-48 hours after perming before coloring.

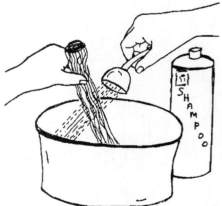

The first time you shampoo the weft, use a deep cleansing shampoo. Towel dry the weft, then apply the color. Color spreads more evenly if the hair is damp.

Remember – Color Pigment Has Been Removed

When you're going to add color to factory lightened wefts, remember that some of the color pigment has been removed from the hair and that you may have to add extra red or yellow pigment to compensate.

Do A Test Strand

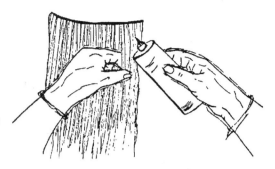

Always, always do a test strand. You need to see if your formula is correct – you need to work out the correct timing. Probably the most common mistake made in coloring is that stylists just go ahead and color or lighten the entire weft. Always do a test strand.

Complete Coverage Is Very Important

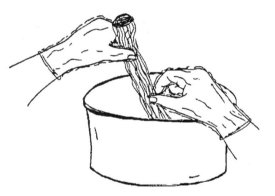

Depending on the space available for you to do your work, adapt your coloring techniques accordingly. If you are going to completely color the weft, use a bowl. Immerse the weft in the color and work it through the hair thoroughly – sort of like kneading bread dough.

Do NOT leave the weft. Because the hair is porous, it will take color quickly. Stay with it. Sometimes the hair can process within 2-5 minutes.

Do NOT place the weft in a plastic bag, or wrap in a towel. Do not put the weft in the hair dryer. All these things can cause uneven distribution.

Lowlighting or Highlighting

If you are lowlighting or highlighting, spread the weft out on a non absorbent surface. The easiest thing to do is to spread out a plastic wrap and put your weft on this.

Foiling a Weft

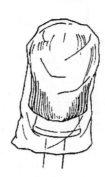

Prepare Manikin Head for Foiling
If you are going to foil the weft, first cover your Manikin head with a plastic bag.

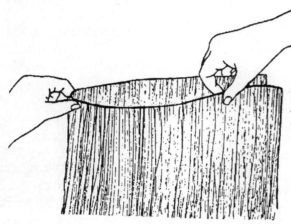

Fold Weft
Just as you did for perming a weft, fold the weft in half.

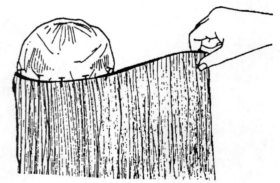

T-pin the Weft to the Manikin Head
Starting above the ear, attach the weft to the head by inserting T-pins into the sewing on the top of the weft. Space the T-pins 2" to 3" apart. If the width of the weft (even folded in half) is greater than the circumference of the head, when you reach the point where you began, T-pin the remaining weft just above the previous row.

Making the Hair Natural Looking

There are a few tricks you can use to make the hair really natural looking. As an example, you can apply one color to one side of the weft, then turn the weft over and apply a slightly different shade.

To match a client's hair that has had some sun-bleaching – you can either highlight or lowlight the hair. Also, you can brush some bleach just on the ends – lightening them up just as the sun would.

Gray and White Hair

Matching gray, very light blonde and white hair is still a problem. It is difficult to lift black Chinese or Indian hair all the way to the very light blonde shades, let alone white. There are only a few choices in dealing with clients with these hair colors.

One solution involves blending white synthetic fiber in with the human hair. Of course you can't perm blended synthetic/human hair.

Another approach that is being tested is using yak hair. In the '60s, yak hair was often used to make inexpensive wigs. The yak is related to the buffalo and is raised in Tibet. The stomach hair of a yak is pure white and will grow as long as 8-10" which means the finished length of a weft made of yak hair can be 6-8". Yak hair can be used for short white or very light blonde hair colors. It is possible to lowlight or reverse-frost yak hair to match any color of grey hair.

For short hair styles of very light blonde, gray or white hair, considering the limitations of the weft's color, another approach is to add hair only for volume in the back of the client's head. This hair can be the dark color of their gray hair, leaving their own hair light in front and possibly coloring their own hair in the crown hair to blend it all together with the color light in front, darker in the crown area and even darker in the back.

Mix-Match

One of the favorite tricks of successful stylists is to mix-match different color wefts – high or lowlighting each of them. As an example, you can use a weft in the medium brown range and highlight it and on the next track up use a weft in the golden blonde or even light blonde range and lowlight it.

All Wefts Are Not Equal

Don't assume because one weft has taken color very evenly and you achieved exactly the color you wanted – that you will get it every time. Wefts have their own personality!

BECOMING AN EXPERT

Becoming an expert in coloring can be relatively easy, certainly a lot of fun, and not very expensive. A suggestion, just as in perming, contact your local beauty supplier and/or a color manufacturer. Learn as much as you can about various product lines. Above all, you need to understand the base of each color you use.

The next step is the real fun part – practice. Purchase some short wefts (usually about 8"). The width of this weft is generally 108". That's a lot of hair to use as practice.

Experiment, practice – whatever you want to call it. In no time you'll have a much better understanding of the exciting things you can do with color on hair extensions!

SUMMARY

An understanding of hair coloring principles and techniques is crucial to the practice of hair extension services. Only 100% human hair that has NOT been dyed at the factory can be successfully decolorized and/or colored. The best way to learn coloring techniques is to practice using hair you can purchase from your hair goods source.

Chapter 7

DESIGNING AND STYLING TECHNIQUES

INTRODUCTION

Designing

Designing styles for hair extension services is something very different from anything you've ever done before! For the first time you are not restricted to the client's own hair – you can create a miracle.

You can preplan the style. However, each style on every client will develop, will evolve on its own as you "build" it.

More times than not you will discover that you'll change your mind at some point as you are going. "Should I add one more track here?" "Well, I don't need quite as much hair here." And so on.

To create a style, to build a style by adding hair, it is extremely important that you go back to basics – to apply the principles of design. This aspect of designing styles will be covered in the next chapter.

Styling

Styling techniques are very important. You can select the best hair, create an excellent curl, match the color perfectly, design a fabulous style – but unless you finish the style correctly – you have not completed your miracle.

There is a lot to learn in this area. And, in truth, this is where I would suggest advanced courses. In this book I'll only cover basics.

SUPPLIES

Manikin and holder	Razor and blades
Needle	Shears (for hair cutting)
Thread	Combs and brushes
Filler fiber	Blow dryer and curling iron
Shears ("working")	Liquid styling tools

DESIGN VARIATIONS

Introduction

You have now learned three different attachment techniques – Braid and Sew, Individual Braiding and Bonding. The next step is to learn how to create the design – the placement pattern for a style. The following are some suggestions.

The Braid/Sew and Bonding techniques require more definition in your placement pattern. The individual braiding technique allows for easier placement patterns in that you can start and stop at almost any point. No matter which technique or combination of techniques you use, it is important to follow a pattern. A defined placement pattern allows for better styling and easier maintenance by you and the client.

Basic 2-Tracks

You will do tracking, whether it's with Braid and Sew, Individual Braiding or Bonding. Remember, it is very important that you always make neat, clean parts. Short hair caught in either your braid or in the bonding is painful and can be pulled out by the roots.

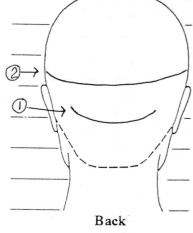

Back

A basic 2-track placement consists of: **Track #1** (the bottom track) starts about 1" above the hairline at the nape of the neck. It is a U-shaped track.

Track #2, also U-shaped, starts 1" in from the hairline and 1" above the ear and follows the contour of the head. This may be all that is needed for a very basic style.

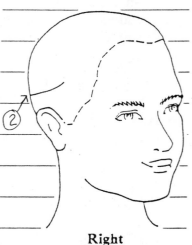

Right

If this is a braided track, you may add a weft double-density, that is, two thicknesses. The best way to do this is to sew one weft on the bottom of the track and then sew the second weft to the top of the track.

If you are bonding the wefts, you can only add one weft at a time. When bonding it is best to only do single-density tracks. For more volume you will need to add more tracks, closer together.

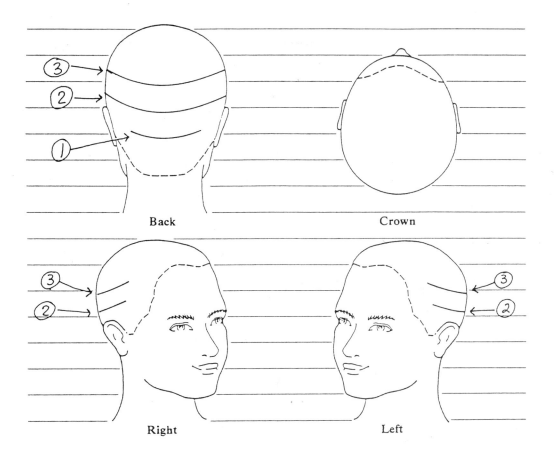

Back   Crown

Right   Left

Basic 3-Tracks

A basic 3-track placement pattern is done similarly to the 2-track technique. You will usually place the tracks a little closer.

Track #1 is at least 1" above the nape hairline. It is U-shaped following the contour of the head.

Track #2 follows the contour of the head and is closer to track #1.

Track #3 again follows the contour of the head.

The 3-track placement pattern is probably the most common. This is usually enough hair to add for volume, for length or for both.

Naturally, if you need 4 or 5 tracks, such as on a bonded style, you would add these a little closer together. As you see, so far you are only working with a basic pattern.

Full Coverage 6-Tracks

Full coverage is when most or all of the client's own hair is covered. There are a lot of variations – far too many to cover in this book.

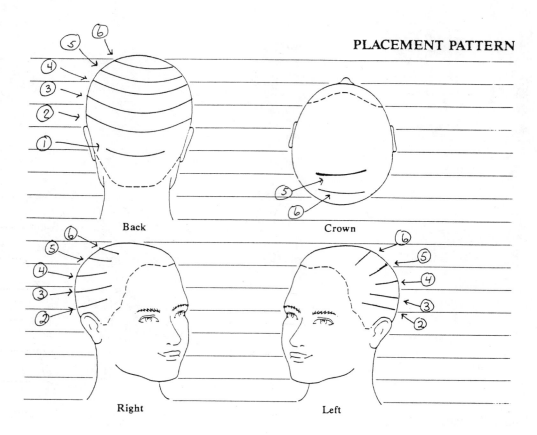

PLACEMENT PATTERN

In this pattern, follow the same procedures for the 3-track pattern shown earlier. Then, for the front and top, add tracks #4, #5 and #6. If you are braiding the tracks, do single braids (instead of two braids toward the center). You usually alternate the braids, braiding #4 from left to right, #5 from right to left, and #6 from left to right.

Be sure to devise ways to keep from having a large clump of hair at the end of the braid. Keep in mind where your client places her/his head when sleeping. A large clump of hair can be uncomfortable. Also be aware of how you are going to include the extra hair at the end of the braid either back over the braid or into the hairstyle.

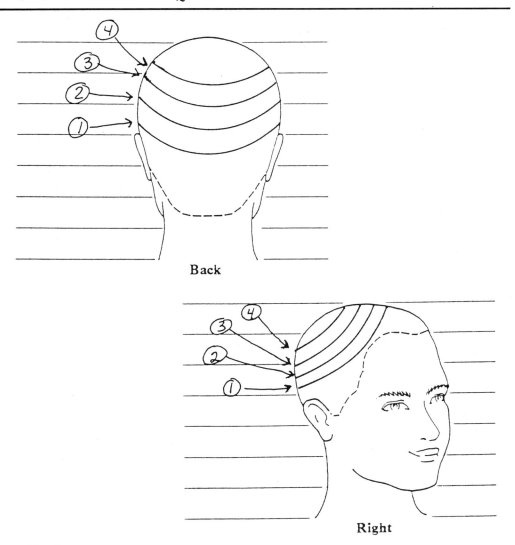

Back

Right

Circular 4-Track

This is a very popular pattern. It allows a lot of coverage with minimal tracking.

Track #1 begin braiding 1" from the hairline above the right ear. This braid goes all the way around – ending where you began. Again, be aware of how you will end this track.

Tracks #2, #3 and **#4** are braided following the contour of the client's head. You can do 2-braid tracks or 1-braid tracks. Just remember, if you do 1-braid tracks be conscious of where you end the braid and what you will do with the hair at the end of the track.

Ordinarily you would not use this pattern for the bonding technique.

Circular for Complete Coverage

This pattern is similar to the 4-track circular pattern, only with more hair. Usually this pattern is used when there will be none of the client's own hair exposed.

Sometimes you will have clients with really special needs. An example of this is one of our models in this book. Leann was eight months pregnant and still working. Her time and physical needs were a little different then than they were eight months earlier.

No way is she going to go without her hair extensions! To accommodate her needs, her placement pattern has been designed so that all of her hair comes from the *top* of her head. This pattern allows for more comfort in sleeping, and it is easier, with less hair to maintain.

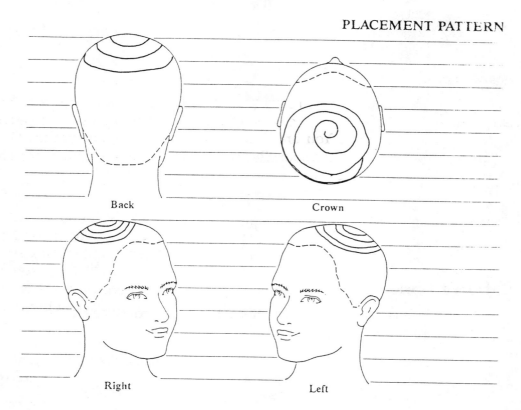

PLACEMENT PATTERN

Back   Crown

Right   Left

The tricky part of this pattern is to determine where the hair will split. You need to work out where the "part" or the "crown" will be placed and how it will be accomplished. If the style is short and curly and can stand up or be back-combed/back-brushed, then the split can be hidden.

DESIGNING AND STYLING TECHNIQUES

Brush-Back/Brush-Up

This is where your imagination, where trial-and-error can play a major part in your creations. Here is an example.

If your client is planning on wearing his/her hair always back or up, you can design the placement pattern accordingly. This is an example of such a pattern. Notice all the tracks are vertical. The hair placed this way is restricted in its styling capabilities, yet it guarantees fullness and/or length where needed for specific styles.

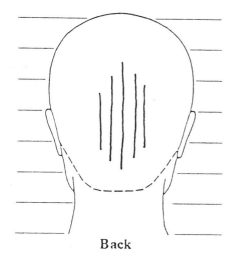
Back

Fashion Fun

For an evening of fun, you can bond in one or more strips of hair. With extra curls, a unique color contrast, etc., all sorts of fun and creative things can be done. You are limited only by your imagination. Of course, remember your responsibilities as to the health of your client's hair, etc.

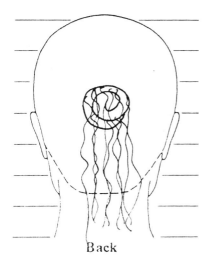
Back

Ponytail (circular)
A ponytail can be created by making a circular track anywhere you'd like to place it. You can also bond strips of wefts or even do large individual braids. What fun!

Ponytail (horizontal)
The placement horizontal placement pattern also works very well when bonding a ponytail style on short hair.

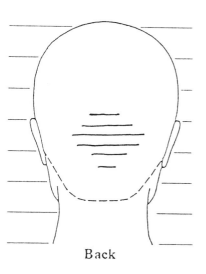
Back

Asymmetrical Design

For a different style, place wefts on one side to create an asymmetrical design. Imagine, your client can go home with a great new look. You can bond, individual braid or micro filler fiber braid in the added hair.

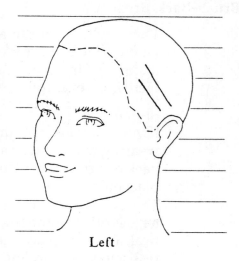

Left

Bangs

Another look, thinning hair — add bangs using any of the three techniques you've learned.

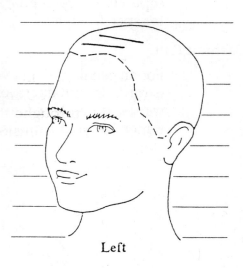

Left

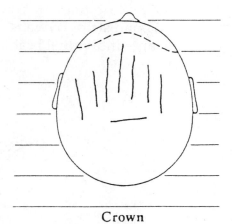

Crown

Volume

With clients who are thinning on top — bond in or do individual braids to add the volume they need.

DESIGNING AND STYLING TECHNIQUES

Color Accents
What fun! Add color without coloring your client's hair. You can use any of the three techniques to add color to your client's hair.

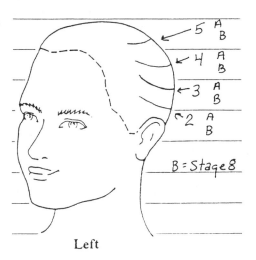
Left

Micro filler fiber braid attachement method would be appropriate for someone who wants color dimension throughout their hair. (See the picture of Kathleen.) Another example would be of a younger person who has ash brown (drab) color hair. Using a stage 8 color wefts throughout would give the hair the illusion of highlighting.

Individual braid method will allow you to give the client long-lasting color accents that will appear as if the hair has been subtly highlighted and/or lowlighted. Or if you want a more dramatic effect, you add more braids of different colors.

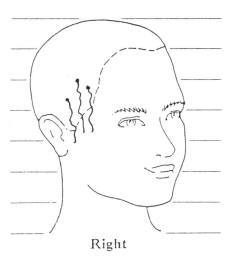
Right

Bonding is an excellent way to *really* have fun for a *special* evening out. Using your imagination you can take some pieces of wefts, color them and bond them in for a real *creation*. Match the client's clothing for the evening with a long curl that matches her dress. Create red and green accents for Christmas parties – be as subtle or as wild as you and your client want!

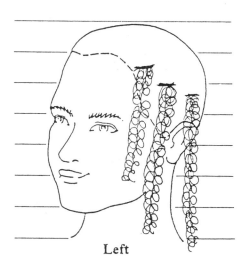
Left

COMBINATIONS

Of course you can combine techniques. One situation in which you might combine braiding and bonding is when the hair in a certain area is not long enough to braid but you want to add hair in this area anyway.

Another combination would be to use track braiding in the back area of the head and individual braids on the sides and front.

I believe that you need to know all three of these basic techniques to be able to accommodate your clientele. Each technique has an application – on its own – or in combination. Just use your imagination – and common sense and you'll be very surprised at what you can create!

CUTTING THE STYLE

Problems Due to Client's Own Hair

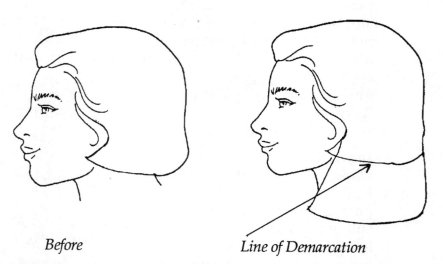

Before   *Line of Demarcation*

When cutting hair extension styles, there are several things to remember. If your client has one-length hair, you cannot just add hair for more length. There will be a line of demarcation. In this case, you will have to either completely cover the client's hair or change the style to a layered look.

Often your client will have really damaged hair. Trying to blend in ends that are in bad shape can be next to impossible. Of course, your client will be resistant to having any of his or her own hair cut to get rid of these ends. This is a problem you are used to dealing with.

Weft Hair Is One Length

The next thing to remember is that the hair in wefts is all one length. This is not how hair grows. As you know, hair on a head is constantly being replaced. As a result, even on one-length hairstyles, the hair is not one length – there are various lengths throughout the head.

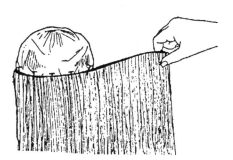

Razor Cut the Added Hair

To accomplish a natural look to the added hair, after it is attached you will need to do a razor cut to the added hair.

Since razor cutting hasn't been used much lately, your client may be very apprehensive when you get the razor out. Be sure to explain what you are doing to the added hair – and why you are doing it.

When doing a razor cut to the added hair, the angle the blade of the razor is held to the hair shaft is the cutting angle.

Heavy Layering – Above 90°

Light Layering – Above 90°

Uniform – 90°

High Graduation – 45° – 90° = High

Low Graduation – 0° – 45°

Solid – 0°

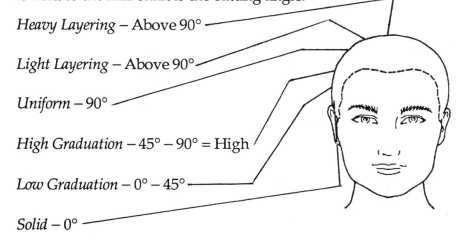

The Cut Is Critical

I have seen hundreds of hair extension styles and probably the one most telling aspect is the cut. It's hard to know exactly what is "not quite right." What it is – is that the hair doesn't really seem to move right.

Probably the one single error most stylists (even some of the very best) make when doing hair extensions is in the cutting. You must remember, that on a head of hair, there are many lengths. Because as the hairs fall out they are replaced and grow out. Also as hair is growing, the longer it gets, the thinner the ends.

So for natural looking hair extensions, you must simulate nature all the way by cutting the added hair so that it moves, reacts and responds as if it were hair growing from your client's head.

CURLING/FINISHING

OK – it's time to use any and all curling and finishing techniques! You can finger wave, pincurl set, roller set, use electric rollers, steam rollers, curling iron, blow dry and any combination of these.

You can use your liquid styling tools also. But remember, if you are using the bonding technique – be sure not to use and warn your client not to use – products with oil.

The most common mistake stylists make is not finishing the style. You have done a great deal of work – be sure to finish the job – be sure to finish the style!

A hairstyle is not a hairstyle until it is finished. Walking out the door is your signature – your name. Finish it!

SUMMARY

Your placement pattern is critical to the overall style – where you add hair determines the basic attributes of the style. You can use any of three methods you have learned, or you can combine them. Where you add hair is restricted only by considerations of the health of the client's hair, the client's lifestyle and how well you can hide the attachment technique. The only other limitation is your imagination!

A hair extension style should be undetectable. A hair extension style is *not a style* until it is *finished!*

Chapter 8

PUTTING IT ALL TOGETHER

INTRODUCTION

One Most Important Attribute

At a conference of the National Association of Accredited Cosmetology Schools (NAACS) there was an interesting meeting recently. One of the programs was a panel comprised of individuals from top management of several salon chains. They discussed with school owners what they felt were skills needed by today's cosmetology school graduates. The major areas the panel members felt needed more emphasis in today's schools were:

Better work habits
Better self-image
Greatly improved communication skills

Of all the issues discussed, improvement in communication skills is the one area that every panel member said was the most needed. As one member put it, "We'll hire a stylist who can communicate, can talk with the client and with other employees and has average skills over a stylist who has excellent skills and little or no ability to communicate."

When I asked more than 100 stylists what they thought were the three most important things to tell other stylists about hair extension services — everyone said that communications with the client was the most important thing. One stylist, Carrie Leger, listed what she thought were the *three* most important things to tell other stylists as:

1. Communicate
2. Communicate
3. Communicate

The Ten Commandments of Human Relations

Hanging on the bulletin board at a local radio station is this document. I think it's very applicable to our business.

1. *Speak to People*
   There is nothing so nice as a cheerful word of greeting.

2. *Smile at People*
   It takes 72 muscles to frown, only 14 to smile.

3. *Call People by Name*
   The sweetest music to anyone's ears is the sound of their own name.

4. *Be Friendly and Helpful*
   If you would have friends, be a friend.

5. *Be Cordial*
   Speak and act as if everything you do is a genuine pleasure.

6. *Be Genuinely Interested in People*
   You can like almost everybody if you try.

7. *Be Generous with Praise*
   Cautious with criticism.

8. *Be Considerate*
   with the feelings of others. There are usually three sides to a controversy; yours, the other fellow's and the right side.

9. *Be Alert*
   to give service. What counts most in life is what we do for others.

10. *Add to This*
    a good sense of humor, a big dose of patience, a dash of of humility and you will be rewarded manyfold.

Author Unknown

Confidentiality

Many years ago I met the woman who was responsible for an ad campaign for Clairol that in those days was resisted because it seemed too risque. Remember "Only your hairdresser knows for sure"? Well, the same thing applies to hair extensions. No one wants to go around and advertise that their hair color is not their own – no one wants to go around and tell everyone that they have hair extensions. As their stylist, you too should respect their feelings. Don't worry, they'll tell their best friends and word of mouth will send you a lot of business. Gossip will, however, give you a bad reputation.

Teamwork

If you are not an expert in all aspects of hair extension services, you might go into partnership with other stylists who can augment your skills. Because there is money involved in hair extension services, this is one area where you might consider teaming up with other stylists. All stylists involved in servicing this client should be involved in the initial consultation. One member of the team needs to be the "director," with the other members of the team as the specialists. Each aspect of hair extension services can be done by different stylists.

Factors to Consider

Pricing hair extension services is different than any other services you have done. There are a number of factors to consider. These include:

Supplies
The supplies you'll use for hair extension services are the same as for any other services with the addition of the hair you are going to add. So this part of costing/pricing is easy. Some stylists and salons treat the hair as a "retail" item that, like wigs, bathing suits, underwear, etc., is not returnable and not refundable.

If your source for hair serves hairstylists exclusively and the hair is of excellent, dependable quality, you can make a profit on the hair in addition to the services. In this book I've used a system of pricing that I believe is one of the more workable ones devised to date. In this case, the hair is marked up and is considered a retail item.

Training
You have invested more in training time and expense than other stylists and that is considered a commodity. The more training you have, the more skills you have, the more you can demand for your services.

Time
Probably the easiest way to calculate your pricing is to work out how much you are charging relative to the time you invest in the service. As an example, take the amount you are charging for a haircut.

If you are doing two haircuts per hour, your hourly income is the amount charged per haircut *times* two. Or, on an average, with all the services you do in the salon, you can *divide* your income by the hours you work. What is your average income per hour?

Because hair extension services are specialized, you should be making at least what you make as an average income, when you first start.

After you have learned more techniques, have become an expert, you should be making *two, three* and even *four* times more than you would doing any other services.

I know many stylists who are making less than $3.00 an hour doing hair extension services. In some cases, these stylists have seriously underestimated their services and their skills. However, some of the work I have seen, no matter what the stylist has charged, isn't worth any more than $3.00 an hour. The reason I say this is simply that many stylists doing hair extensions just don't learn all the things they need to know. Hair extensions that are worth the money – and the time – are those which are healthy (safe) for the client's own hair and are natural-looking. All aspects of the services must be done completely – curling, cutting, coloring and adding hair!

Record Keeping

It is rather obvious that record keeping for your hair extension clients is probably more important than for any other type of client. You have a lot to keep track of. Sometimes your client will call and will want "fresh" hair – so without having the client come in, you'll have to reorder hair and maybe service it.

And, above all, you'll need to do follow-up telephone calls to your clients. See how everything is going for them. Maybe they are not returning because of a financial problem. Maybe you can work out a way to do maintenance in smaller increments more frequently.

Record keeping can also keep you protected for any possible "sue-happy" clients. It's too bad, but nowadays we have to protect ourselves all the time. It seems that a lot of people need someone else to blame instead of being responsible for their own actions. So, record keeping is just good business – both for positive and possible negative situations. Protection and Profits!

Organizing Time

Scheduling Time and Services
Scheduling your time for hair extension services can be difficult. If you are already working a full book, then it might be very difficult for you to make the necessary changes.

Most successful stylists doing hair extensions are either ones who are just starting out in an area and did not have a large clientele, or ones who were ready for a complete change and decided to lose some of their current clients for new hair extension clients. It's a tough decision sometimes – but you can't do it all.

Consultation Time
The first thing you must schedule is time for a consultation with your prospective client. You'll need forms, pen/pencil, a place where you can talk, your usual tools (combs, etc.) and a mirror. It also helps if you have a Manikin that you have already prepared to demonstrate the various techniques you use so the prospective client can observe how each technique is done. Naturally, you'll want to show the client some hair, so you client can see and feel it. And display some pictures of styles. Your consultation time should be 30-60 minutes. If you charge a fee for your consultations, you should charge whatever you would be making on an average for this period of time.

Client's Own Hair Services
I have never heard of a client who didn't want hair extensions right then – that minute! But it's not possible. First you need to book time to service your client's own hair. It's advisable to do all required chemical services ahead of time – while you're waiting for the hair to arrive. One way to best service your customer is – first do any perming or straightening services required. On later appointments, do any coloring required.

Order and Prepare Wefts

One of the wonderful things about hair extension services is that you do not have to maintain any inventory. You collect a deposit from the client, which should cover the cost of the hair and the cost of any services you plan to do to the weft. Sometimes clients will change their mind later, but at least you've collected the deposit and explained that it's not refundable because you have had to make an investment in hair and in services on the hair!

Attachment and Styling

Next you must schedule time for attaching, cutting and styling. Depending on the technique you are going to use, how much hair you'll be adding, etc., you may need to schedule anywhere from two hours to 14 hours. Remember, your time is money. Don't undersell yourself!

Follow-Up Services

I really recommend the free check-up appointment, about one week to twelve days after you have done your client's extensions. During this visit, you will check to see how well the attachments are staying in, the condition of the client's scalp (any rashes or hot spots developing?) – and the condition of the client's hair and the added hair. Is the client taking proper care of the hair? Cleaning properly? Conditioning properly?

This 15-20 minute visit can save you many a sad story and bad publicity. It also is a way of "bonding" with your client. You really care how things are going and your client will know it.

SUPPLIES

General

- Pencil
- Tape measure
- Manikin with extensions
- Hairstyle picture book(s)
- Camera (optional)
- Comb
- Weft samples
- Hair color picture book
- Calculator
- A quite place

Forms

- Client file folder
- *Consultation Work Sheet* – Figure 1-4
- *Services Price Sheet* – Figure 5
- *Hair Costing Sheet* – Figure 6
- *Hair Pricing Sheet* – Figure 7
- *Chemical Services Release Form* – Figure 8
- *Hair Extension Agreement* – Figure 9
- *Model's Agreement/Release Form* – Figure 10
- *Hair Extension Release Form* – Figure 11
- *Chemical Services Record Form* – Figure 12
- *Home Care Instructions* – Figure 13

CONSULTATION OBJECTIVES

Introduction

Now that you have learned your attachment techniques and have boned up on perming and coloring – this is where you will set the tone for your success. The consultation with a prospective hair extension client is the most important part of your relationship. This is where any problems can be solved before they become problems!

The reason for a consultation includes the following objectives:

Establish Relationship
The consultation is a way to establish the basis of your relationship with the client. This relationship, of course, depends on the type of person you are and the type of person the client is. Primarily, your client (prospective client) has come to you, the expert, to solve a problem for her or him. This does not make you a "superior" person – but rather a person with knowledge and skill.

Determine Client's Needs
You will need to determine, first, what the clients want and need. Sometimes their wants are not the same as, from your professional viewpoint, what their needs are. If there is a big gap between their wants and needs, you'll have to make some decisions. As an example someone may want long, long hair, and you feel that this is not the right style for this person. What do you do? (We'll discuss this later.)

Evaluate All Factors
You will need to evaluate all nineteen factors of the *Consultation Work Sheet (Figures 1 and 2)*. This information will help you determine what needs to be done to the client's own hair and to the hair to be added.

Advise Client of Commitment
It is very important that you advise your client of exactly what is involved in hair extension services. First, what will be required for the initial servicing, time and costs and techniques. Second, what is involved in maintenance – at home and for in-salon up keep. *(Consultation Work Sheet, Figures 3 and 4.)* Both need to be explained in terms of time and money to the client. There should never be any surprises when it comes to how much time and money is involved initially and from then on.

Determine Advisability
You must also determine if this is a client *you want* to service. Not only does the client have an investment, but you do too. Your time, your skills and your reputation are all involved. If you think that this client will not properly care for the hair – then don't be greedy – don't take the business. This kind of client will cause you more grief in the long run.

Candida

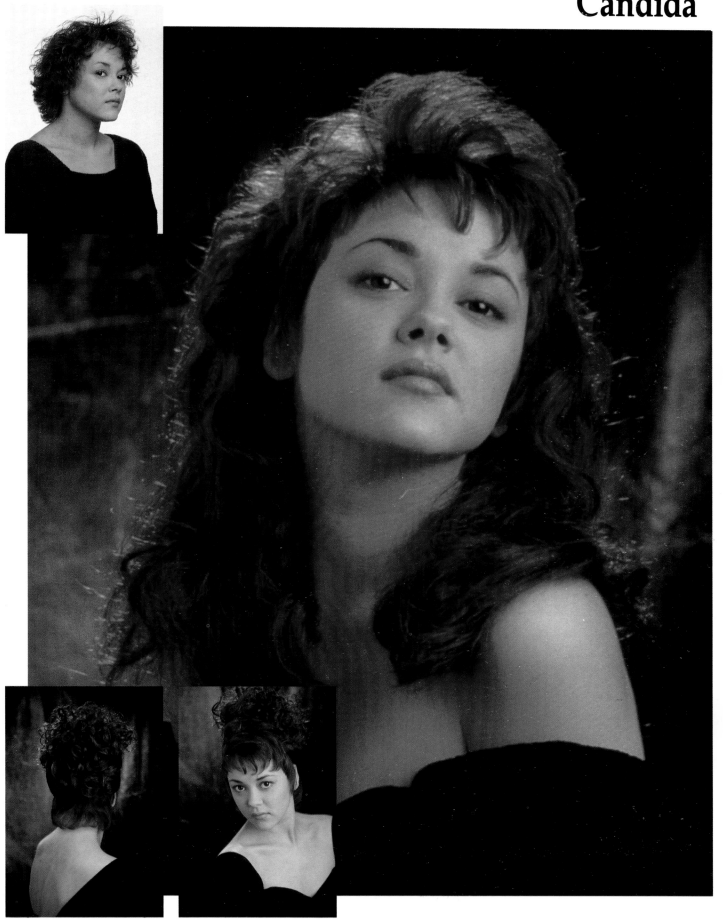

Ramin

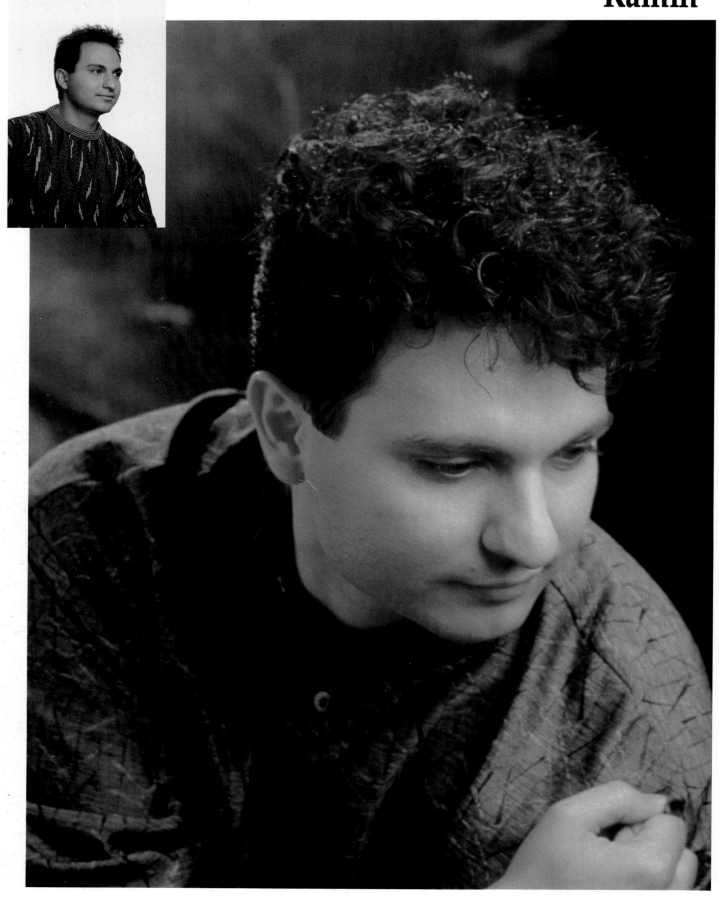

Arlene

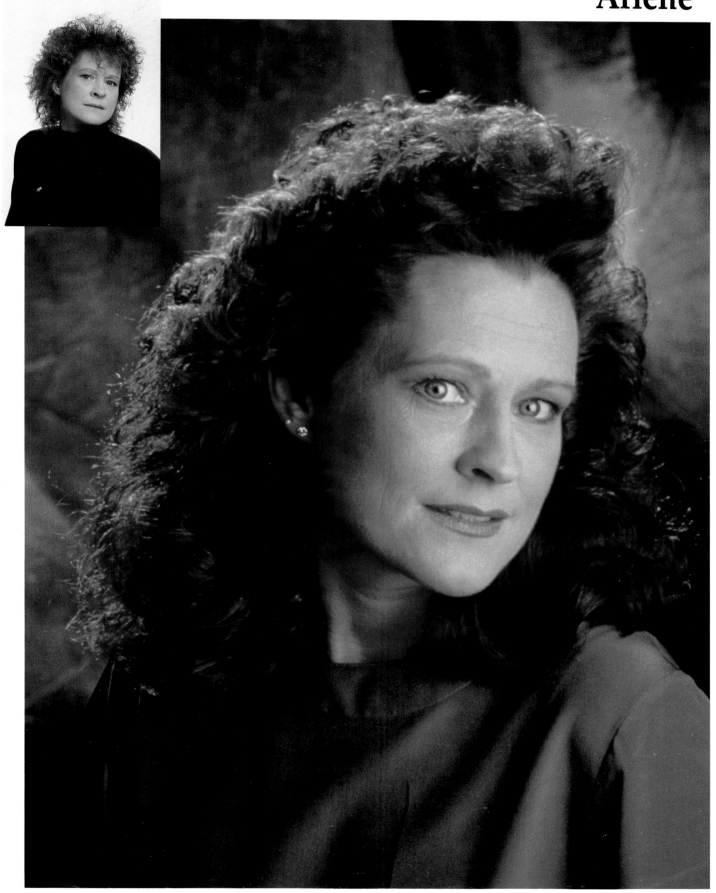

Leann

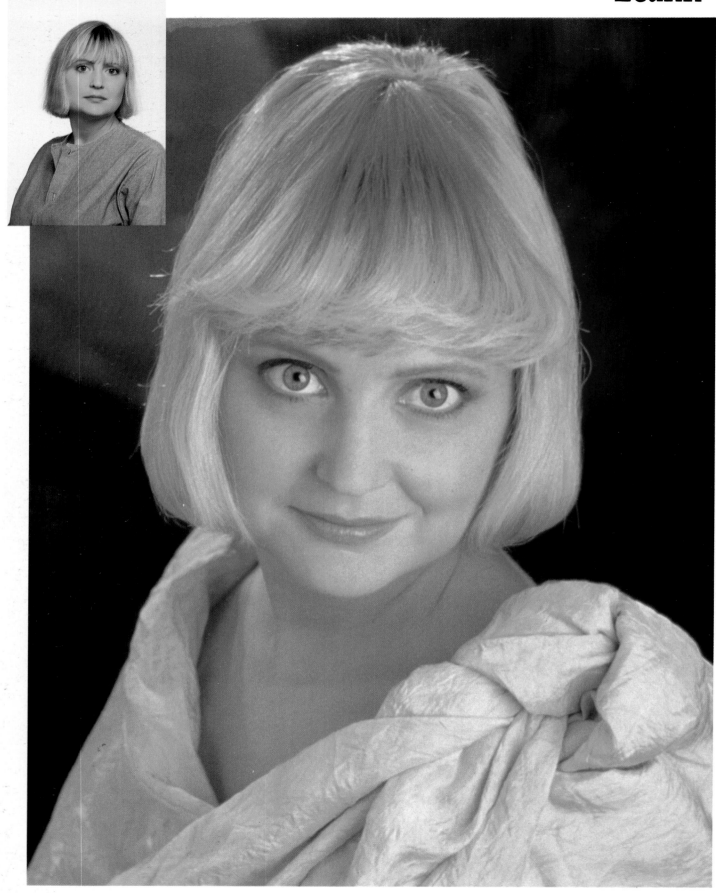

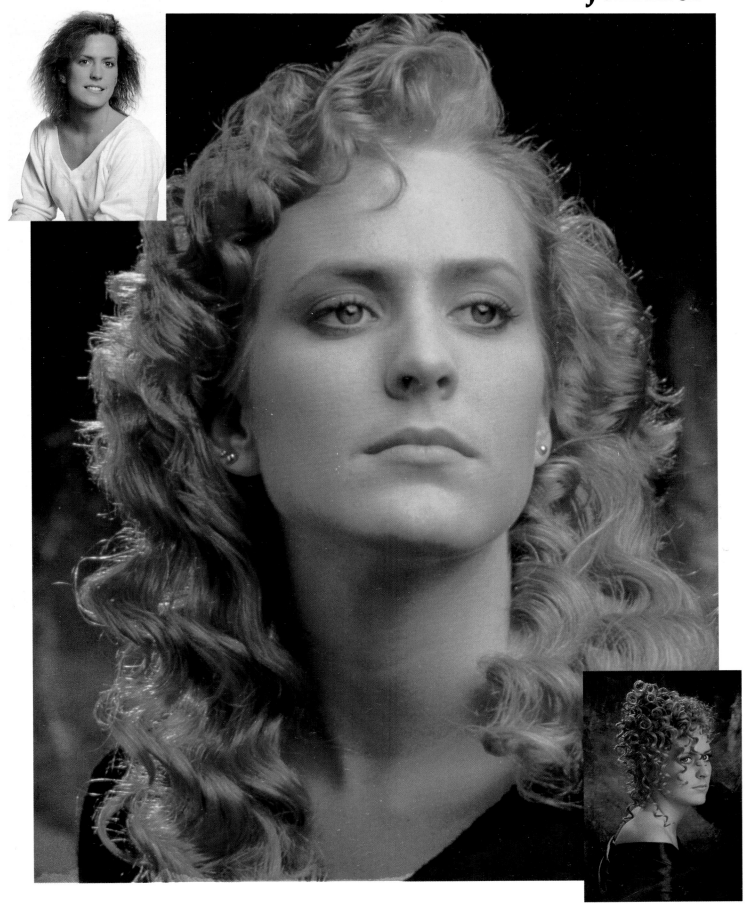

Jennifer

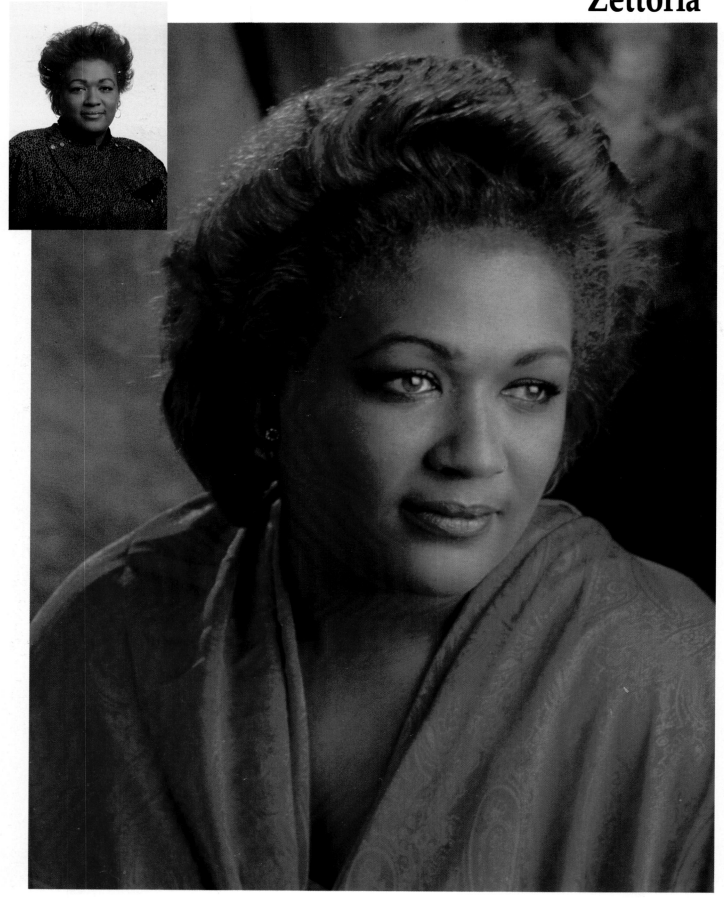

Zettoria

Wanda

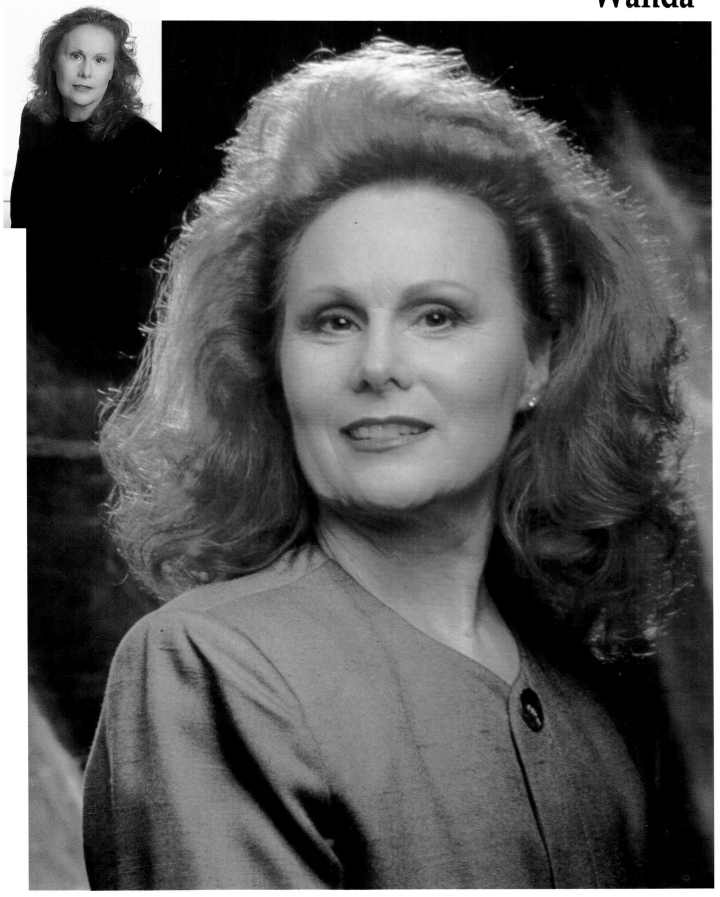

Lynn

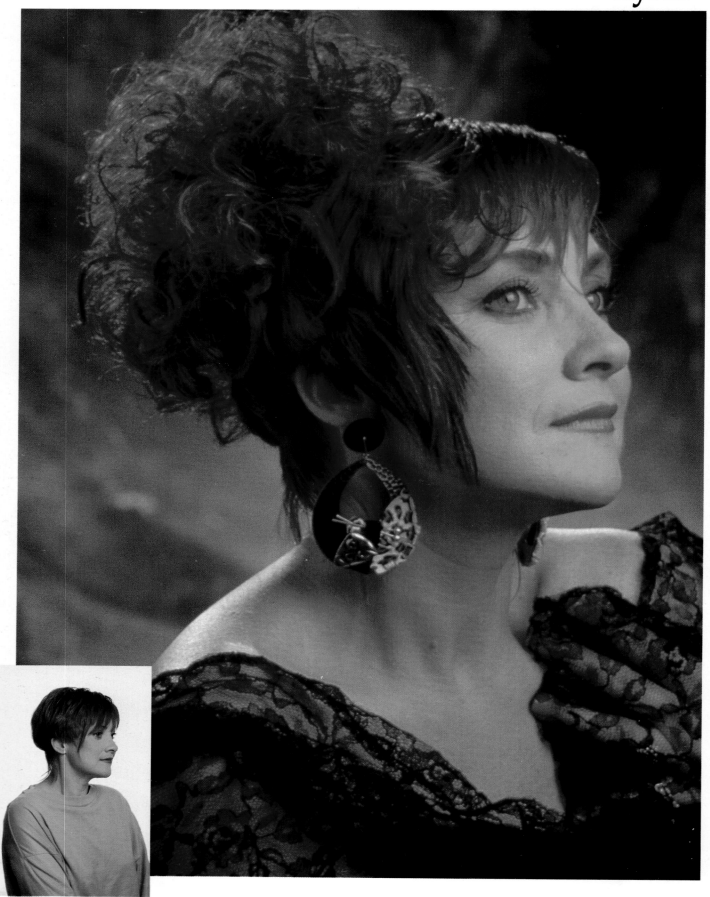

Alondra

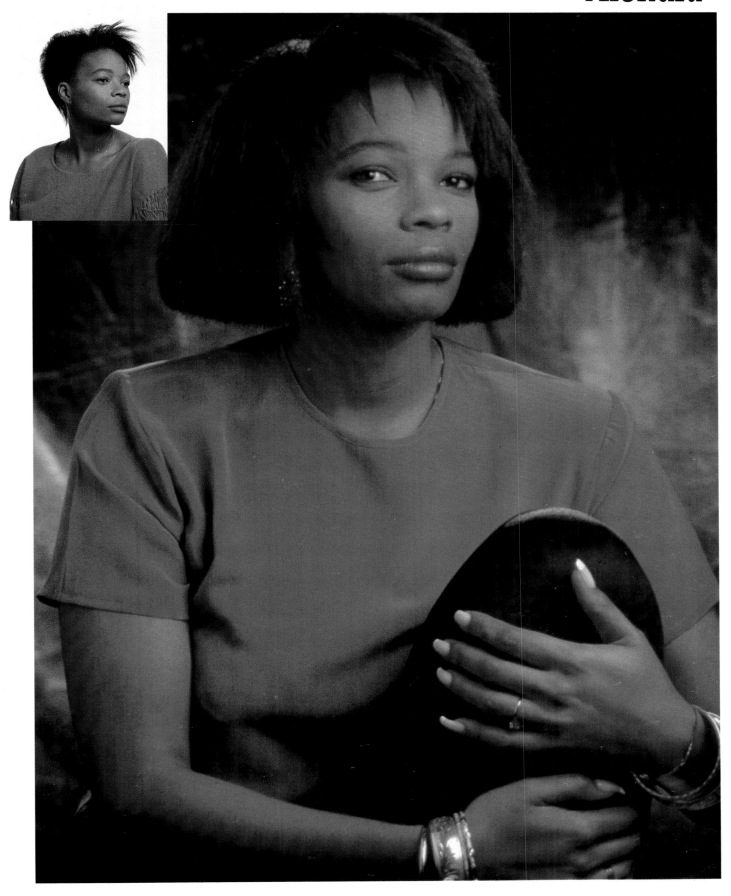

Dana

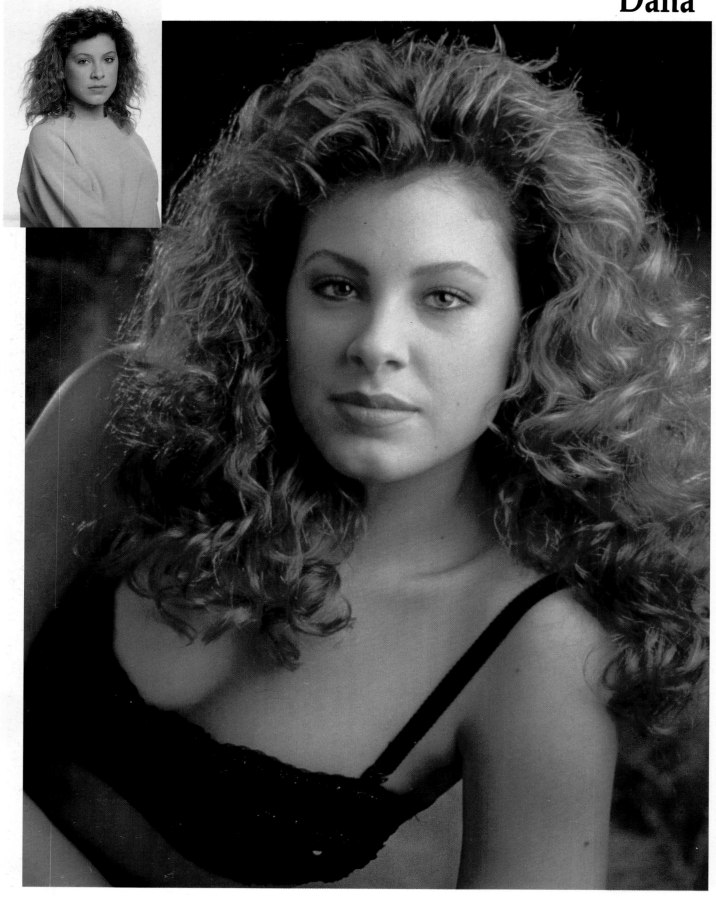

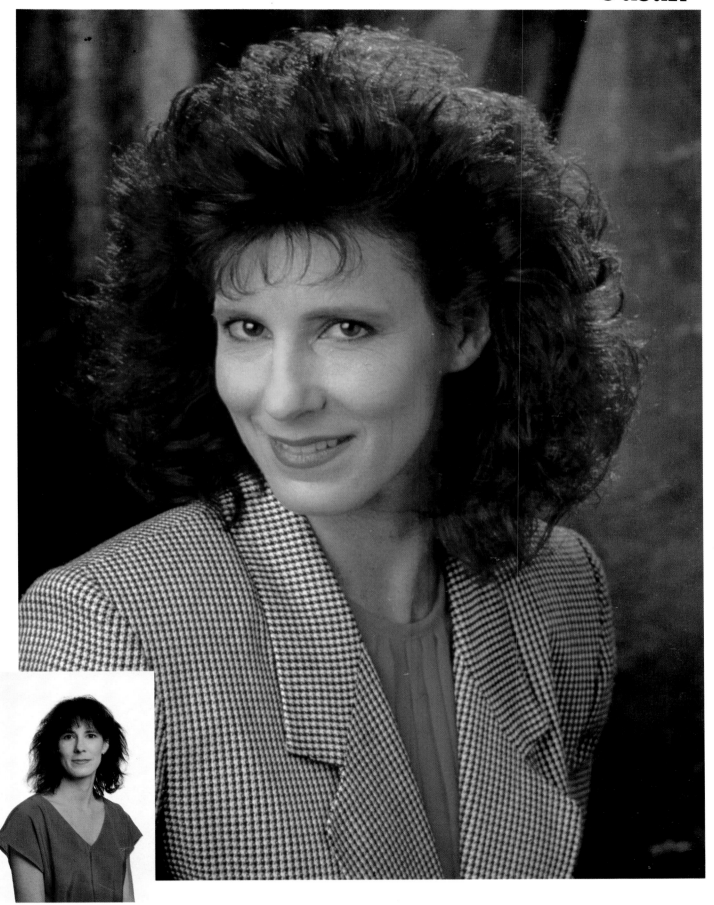

Susan

Larry

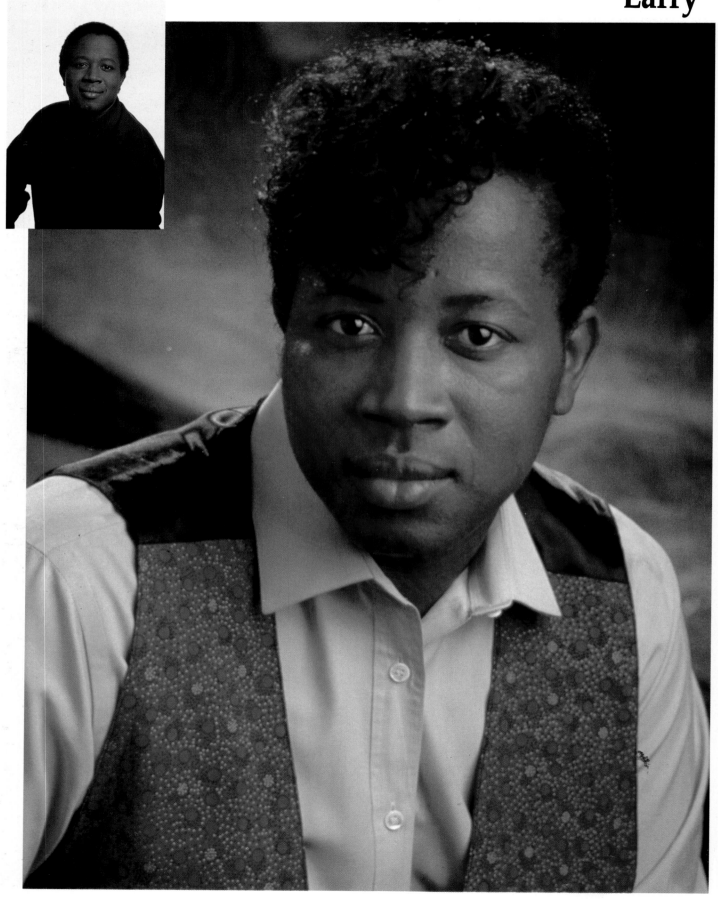

Erin

Janice

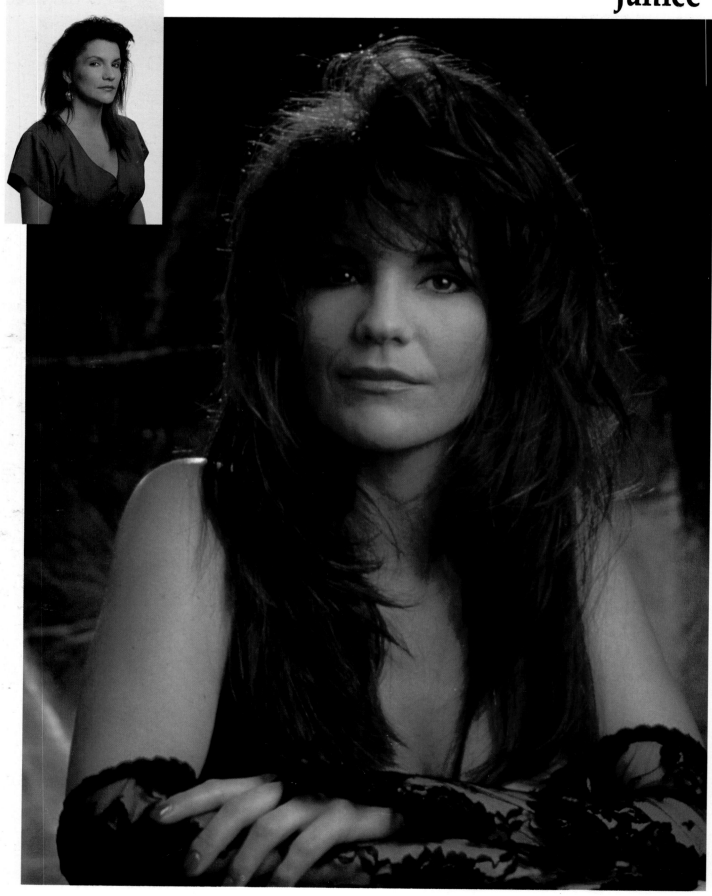

Kathleen

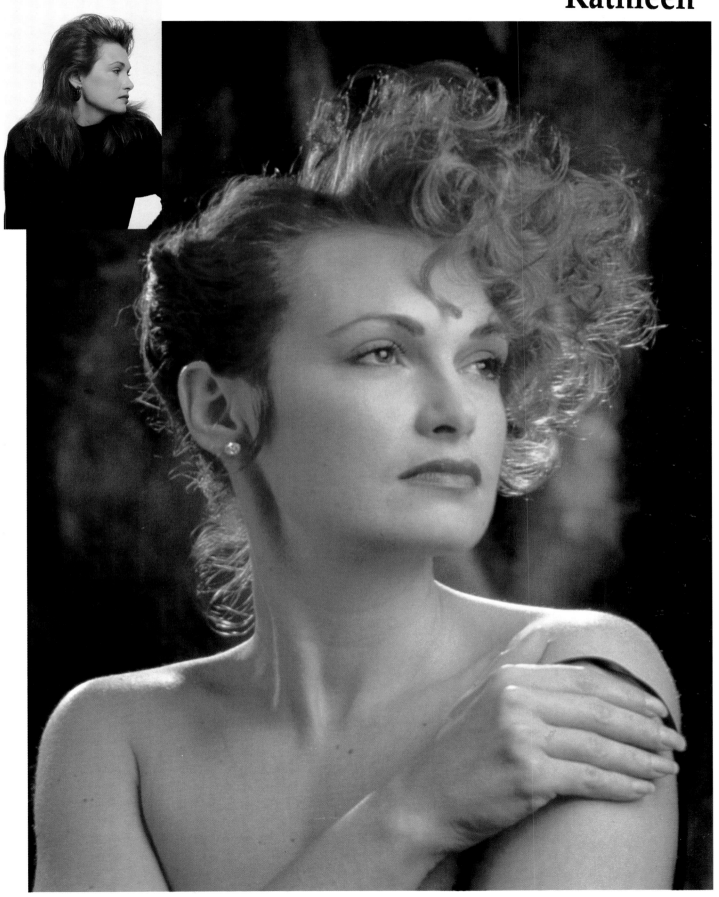

Marla

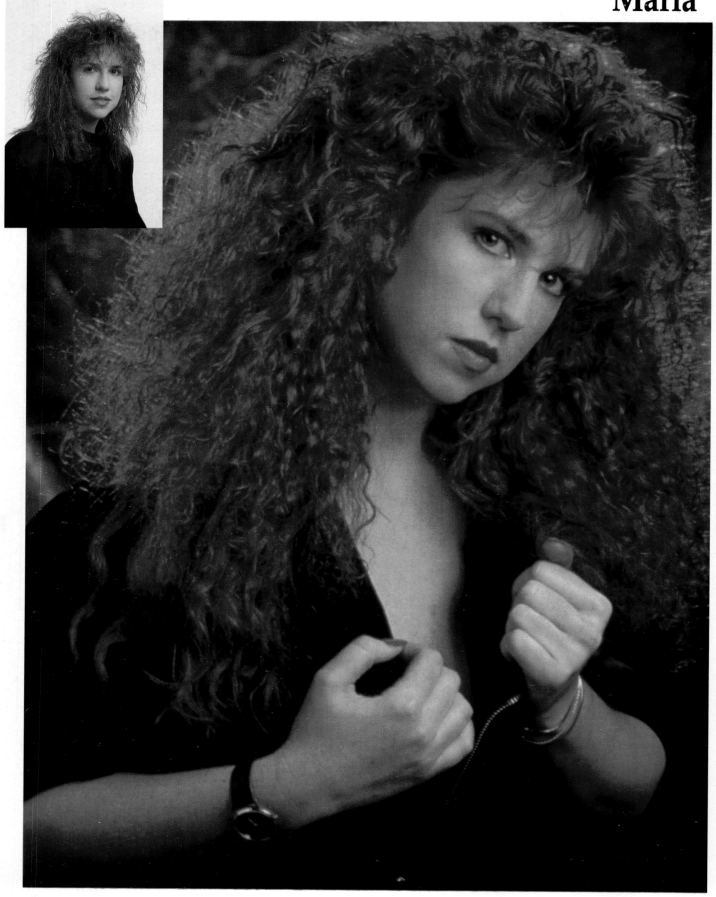

PUTTING IT ALL TOGETHER

Get a Commitment

A commitment has to be made by the client. The logical way is to have them make a deposit. As a matter of fact, you should never do a new client without a deposit. You will have an investment before you even service that client. You need to purchase the hair, process that hair, and reserve time on your book (refuse other business). So, before you begin, your client has to say "yes" by making a deposit.

Many stylists doing hair extension services charge a fee for their consultation time (30-60 minutes). Usually they apply this fee toward the charges of the hair extension service. You may need to consider doing this, because you'll find a lot of your time may be taken up with consultations. You can reduce the number of lookie-lou's by charging for the consultation. If you decline doing the client, or the client decides not to have it done, some stylists refund the deposit. Others keep it as compensation for work they could have been doing during that time or apply it to other services.

Be Prepared

Hair Color Picture Book

When preparing for your consultation – be prepared! A hair color picture book is a very helpful tool. It never is advisable to use hair color manufacturer's color charts when discussing hair colors. Make a hair color book by cutting out pictures from magazines. You then put them together in groups by colors, with dividers inbetween each group of colors. When your clients say, "I'd like red hair," you can find the red *they mean*.

Hairstyle Picture Books

Hairstyle books are a *must!* Your clients are going to change their looks and you need some books to help guide them. The hairstyle books don't have to be specifically ones dealing with hair extensions – its the finished look you are seeking.

CONSULTATION WORK SHEET

Introduction

The *Consultation Work Sheet* has taken years of development. It is my pleasure to share it with you. The following pages will "walk" you through each section of this work sheet.

When designing a hair extension style, the client's hair texture, density and length are obvious considerations. You need to determine how much of their own hair will be a part of their style. Are you going to match the texture? Change their hair texture? Do a complete cover-up so none of the client's own hair is exposed? Do you need to add volume (density) as the basic style design – or only as a balance to the length you are adding? Is the length of the client's hair going to cause any problems relative to attachment techniques or styling versatility?

These kinds of questions are relatively straightforward but need to be discussed with your clients so they are aware of what you are considering as you create their new look.

First you will get all the basic information, such as name and address, phone numbers and the month and day of their birthday. (You can use the client's birthday, for PR – that is give them a special birthday discount, send a birthday card.)

HAIR EXTENSION SERVICES – Consultation Work Sheet

Name: _____ Date: _____
Address: _____ Work #:(___)_____
City
State & Zip: _____ Home #:(___)_____
Stylist: _____ Birthday: _____

1. Reason for Extensions:

2. Life Style: (work and recreation)

3. Home Care Habits: (frequency and products)

Shampooing _____

Conditioning _____

Set and Styling Tools and Products _____

Chemical Work Done at Home _____

4. Salon Habits: (frequency and products)

Shampooing _____

Conditioning _____

Cut and Finish _____

Permanent Waving _____

Color _____

Extensions _____

Other _____

5. Stature:
☐ Large
☐ Medium
☐ Petite

6. Hair Condition:
☐ Dry
☐ Oily
☐ Bleached
☐ Tinted
☐ Normal

7. Hair Texture:
☐ Coarse
☐ Medium
☐ Fine
☐ Very Fine

8. Hair Porosity:
☐ Good
☐ Moderate
☐ Poor
☐ Extremely Porous
☐ Resistant
☐ Build-Up

9. Hair Elasticity:
☐ Poor
☐ Normal
☐ Good

10. Hair Density:
☐ Thick
☐ Medium
☐ Thin

11. Hair Form:
☐ Straight
☐ Wavy
☐ Curly
☐ Extra Curly
☐ Permed

12. Scalp Condition:
☐ Good
☐ Abrasions
☐ Loose
☐ Tight
☐ Oily
☐ Dry
☐ Balding

13. Hair Length:
Front _____
Right _____
Left _____
Crown _____
Back _____

14. Desired Length:
Front _____
Right _____
Left _____
Crown _____
Back _____

15. Hair Color:
Natural   Faded
Streaked   % Gray
_____
_____

16. Sensitive to:
List types of products
_____
_____
_____
_____

© Copyright 1990 Garland Drake International ®   Used with permission from Garland Drake International ®   1207/GDIF01

Figure 1 – Page 1 of 4

PUTTING IT ALL TOGETHER

1. Reason for Extensions:

The reason this prospective client desires to have hair extensions is important for you to know. Just before going on a vacation is not a good time to have extensions done. The reason you should not do extensions for the first time on a client who is going on vacation is that this is no time for the client to be concerned with, or to learn, how to care for the hair!

Evaluate the client's reasons. Are they realistic? You may stop your consultation right here and avoid problems later on.

However, if you believe that the client's reasons are valid, are achievable – then proceed to the next question.

2. Life Style: (work and recreation)

When creating any style for a client, life style is always a consideration. This is even more important when adding hair. You need to be aware of issues such as daily exercising with the need for daily shampooing, time available for caring for a style, and so on.

> You need to ask your clients what kind of work they do.
> What hobbies?
> What sports?

The reason for these questions is to help you determine if the client has the kind of life style that will accommodate the care necessary to hair extensions. People with very active life styles may simply not have the necessary time required. People who are physically active may have other potential problems – such as rashes caused by perspiration caught in the tracks, etc.

The bonding technique may not be advisable for people who must wash their hair daily. In this case, braided tracks or individual braids are probably better. If the client has a lot of hair and does not want to walk around with wet hair – then the individual braiding technique is best because the hair will dry faster without the bulk of the braid and the thickness of the top of the weft. Or, you may use a combination of braided tracks and individual braids.

Then there are clients who have very busy schedules and virtually no time to dedicate to their hair. Hair extensions for volume can simplify their lives. A style will stay in for a full week and require only styling – brushing or combing in the morning. Any of the three attachment techniques are applicable for this type of client.

3. Home Care Habits: (frequency and products)

This information is important for you to have so that you can guide your consultation and properly teach your client about home care for hair extension services. Ask the following questions:

Does the client color his/her own hair?
Does the client use professional products or drug-store products?
Does the client shampoo daily, weekly?
Does the client perm/straighten his/her own hair?

Remember, if the clients can't correctly care for their own hair, it may be very difficult for them to care for extensions.

4. Salon Habits: (frequency and products)

Like home care habits, a client's salon habits will guide you as to the type of hair extension client this person will be. If this client is a "weekly" – any problems will be minimized. If this client seldom seeks professional hair care, chances are there will be more problems.

If this is a new client for you, you need to know what types of services and products have been used before. What is currently used on the hair?

5. Stature:

When a client comes to you for hair extensions and wants length, you have to be the responsible person – you are the professional. Does your client have shoulders wide enough to carry the desired length? Does your client have the height?

Check the appropriate box or boxes on the form. Remember, in all cases you may check more than one box.

5. Stature:
☐ Large
☐ Medium
☐ Petite

6. Hair Condition:

This is part of your pre-perm, pre-color, pre-extension analysis. Check the appropriate box or boxes.

6. Hair Condition:
☐ Dry
☐ Oily
☐ Bleached
☐ Tinted
☐ Normal

7. Hair Texture:

The texture of your client's hair will help you determine attachment technique(s), hair perming/coloring needs and styling needs. Check the appropriate box or boxes.

7. Hair Texture:
☐ Coarse
☐ Medium
☐ Fine
☐ Very Fine

8. Hair Porosity:

Porosity is important when considering the perming/coloring needs of your client's own hair. Check the appropriate box or boxes.

Before proceeding with hair extension services, you may need to perm or color and/or condition the client's own hair. If your client has build-up of product or medications you may need to give the hair special treatment.

8. Hair Porosity:
☐ Good
☐ Moderate
☐ Poor
☐ Extremely Porous
☐ Resistant
☐ Build-Up

9. Hair Elasticity:

Important if you are going to do any chemical services to the client's hair. Also important for evaluation of the health of your client's own hair.

10. Hair Density:

One of the reasons clients want/need hair extensions is that they want more volume, more density.

11. Hair Form:

One of the reasons your client may want/need extensions has to do with their hair form. Do they want to change it? Do they want to match it?

12. Scalp Condition:

This is very important to check – and to share the information with your client. Naturally if the client's scalp is oily you cannot do the bonding attachment technique. If there are abrasions you may have to deal with this problem before doing any services for the client. If there are any bald areas, be sure to point these out to the client. (You will also mark these on item #17 of the Work Sheet.) It is not only informative for you and your client – but discussing and making complete notes on bald areas can save a lot of trouble in the future!

13. Hair Length:

Here you will measure and note the client's current hair length. First, you'll want to evaluate how much longer you will be making the hairstyle. Also, this is often very interesting information because almost always the client's own hair will appear to be growing more. It will get longer faster because the hair extensions will often protect it from chemical, environmental and external abuse.

14. Desired Length:

At this time in your consultation, you will be working out only approximate lengths. One thing to remember is that most people who want hair extensions want more hair, usually more hair than they need. That is, hair that is too long for them to handle or too long for their stature or their shape of face. One of your jobs will be to encourage your client to accept your professional advice on the proper length of hair.

---

9. Hair Elasticity:
- ☐ Poor
- ☐ Normal
- ☐ Good

10. Hair Density:
- ☐ Thick
- ☐ Medium
- ☐ Thin

11. Hair Form:
- ☐ Straight
- ☐ Wavy
- ☐ Curly
- ☐ Extra Curly
- ☐ Permed

12. Scalp Condition:
- ☐ Good
- ☐ Abrasions
- ☐ Loose
- ☐ Tight
- ☐ Oily
- ☐ Dry
- ☐ Balding

13. Hair Length:
Front_____
Right_____
Left_____
Crown_____
Back_____

14. Desired Length:
Front_____
Right_____
Left_____
Crown_____
Back_____

Particularly if your client *does not* have good home care habits, you may need to encourage your client to *start* with shorter hair. Then, if the extensions are cared for, tell your client that you will consider giving them longer hair the next time.

15. Hair Color:

What is the client's current hair color? Natural? Faded? Streaked? What percentage of Gray? When you are doing hair extension services, often you are doing corrective coloring and make-overs. You are really put to the test many times.

Another alternative you have with hair extensions is that you can do total coverage, which allows you to make a complete color change. Or you may add color to a client's hair with individual braids instead of chemicals.

15. Hair Color:
Natural   Faded
Streaked   % Gray

16. Sensitive to:
List types of products

16. Sensitive To:

Questions on this subject can save you a lot of grief in the future. Unfortunately we live in a society where people want to blame others for their actions/decisions. Since hair extension services are expensive, one of the things that clients will try is to get their money back if they are not happy.

In 99% of the cases I've heard about, the reasons stated by the clients have been unreal, even untruthful. I'll go into these later in this chapter. However, an important issue is sensitivity or allergic reaction. There is no way anyone can be allergic to 100% human hair. However, some people are sensitive or allergic to perm solutions and ingredients in some hair care products. Be sure to ask clients if they are sensitive to adhesive bandages. This could mean they are sensitive to latex (the main ingredient in an adhesive bond). Ask these questions and if in doubt, do patch tests.

17. Growth Patterns:

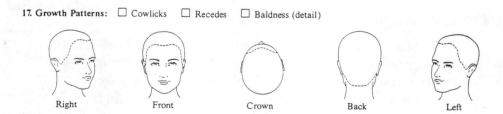

The hair growth pattern on a client's head does affect the work you will be doing. As an example, for individual braid placement, you have to avoid making braids close to a strong cowlick because the hair will separate at that point, exposing the braids. At the same time, placement of a braided track or bonding a weft in an area below a strong cowlick will create the same kind of problem. The hair will separate and expose the weft.

Even more difficult, the reason you are doing hair extension services for this client may be because of a strong cowlick which causes the hair to separate. If you are trying to add hair in an area that is thin or has strong cowlicks, you need to be exceptionally creative. The client has to have enough of their own hair to cover any attachments you've made – unless you have done total coverage. Mark the heads on the *Consultation Work Sheet* accordingly.

17. **Growth Patterns:** ☐ Cowlicks ☐ Recedes ☐ Baldness (detail)

Right   Front   Crown   Back   Left

18. **Facial Shape:**

Oval   Round   Square   Oblong

Pear   Inverted Triangle   Triangle   Diamond   Heart

19. **Head Shape:**

Oval   Narrow Flat   Flat Crown   Pointed hollow nape   Flat Top   Small

Notes:_____

© Copyright 1990 Garland Drake International ®   Used with permission from Garland Drake International ®   1207/GDIF01

Figure 2 – Page 2 of 4

18. Facial Shape:

As you know, there are nine facial types. You need to keep your client's facial type in mind when designing a new look.

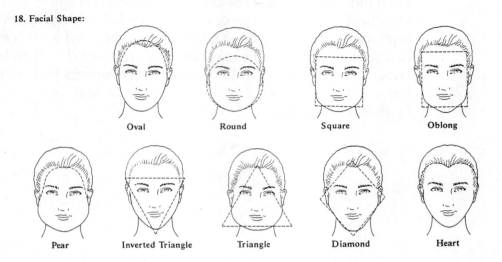

18. Facial Shape:

Oval, Round, Square, Oblong, Pear, Inverted Triangle, Triangle, Diamond, Heart

Oval: The oval face, generally accepted as the perfect face, is about 1 1/2 times longer than its width across the brow and the forehead is slightly wider than the chin. This type of facial shape can wear any style since there are no features to minimize.

Round: For clients with a round face, round hairline and round chin line, your objective is to create the illusion of length to the face. Height on the top of the head, coverage over the ears and part of the cheeks with bangs to one side will reduce the roundness.

Square: The square face has a straight hairline and a square jawline. You can create the illusion of length by styling the hair with a lift off the forehead, moving hair forward at the sides and jaw to add softness and a narrowness to the face.

Oblong: An oblong face is long and narrow with hollow cheeks. Your objective is to make the face appear shorter and wider by styling fairly close to the top of the head with bangs cutting into the forehead and fullness on the sides.

Pear: The client with a narrow forehead, wide jaw and chin line needs to have the illusion created of a wider forehead. Again, height in the front and crown area with the forehead partially covered. A soft wave over the lower jawline can counterbalance this shape of face.

Inverted Triangle: The client with a very narrow forehead, wide jaw and chin line needs to have the illusion created of a wider forehead. Again, height in the front and crown area with the forehead partially covered is needed.

Triangle: The client with a wide forehead and narrow chin line requires a style that increases the width in the chin line and reduces the width of the forehead.

Diamond: The diamond-shaped face is characterized by a narrow forehead, wide cheekbones and narrow chin. You can reduce the width across the cheekbone line by increasing the fullness across the forehead and at the jawline. By styling hair so that it is close to the head at the cheekbone line you can help create the illusion of an oval face.

Heart: A client with a wide forehead and narrow chin line has the heart-shaped face which requires a style that increases the width in the lower part of the face and decreases the width of the forehead. This can be accomplished by using a center part with the bangs rolling away from the face or bangs to one side. In addition, you'll add width and softness at the jawline.

19. Shape of Head:

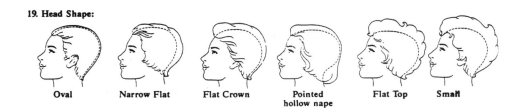

19. Head Shape: Oval, Narrow Flat, Flat Crown, Pointed hollow nape, Flat Top, Small

In addition to your client's facial shape, you need to consider the shape of the head, length of the neck and other features that can be emphasized or minimized.

There are six shapes of heads. For each shape you will want to consider your placement patterns accordingly. In addition to hair styling to accommodate the shape of head, you can add hair to the areas that need more fullness. The oval head is considered the perfect head shape.

Notes:

Here you will write, in detail, things that you really need to remember. This would include any important notes about baldness, hair problems, life style activities that may influence the attachment or care of the extensions, and so on. Consider your client's other facial features. Is the profile straight, or is there a prominent chin, receding forehead, prominent nose, receding chin or protruding chin?

This is a good time to show your client your style books and discuss appropriate and attractive styles. In addition, you can also discuss hair colors using your hair color picture book. (See Chapter 6.)

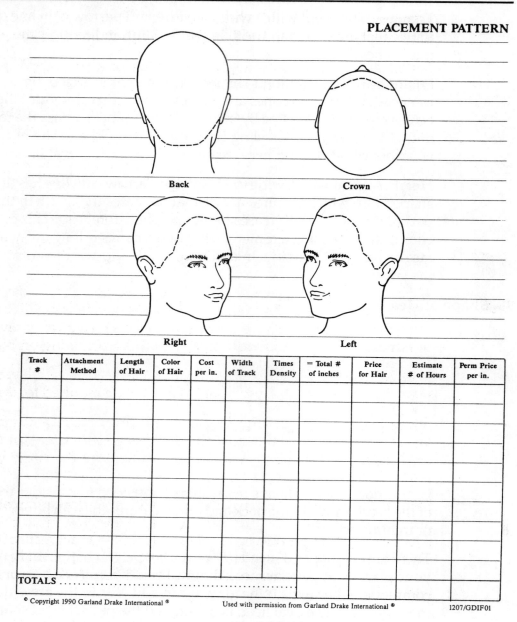

Figure 3 – Page 3 of 4

Placement Pattern

The top portion of this page is where you will draw the tracks, the design, for the client's hair extensions. This is called the placement pattern.

Under the heads there is the area where you work out exactly what you will be doing on each track.
(See *Chapter 7 Designing and Styling Techniques* and *Chapter 9 Case Studies*.)

Track Number On the heads, you draw in the tracks numbering them from the bottom up. *Always building the style* from the bottom up. Under this column then write in the track number placing #1 on the top line.

Attachment Method Indicate whether the hair to be added is done by Braid and Sew (B&S), Individual Braiding (IB) or Bonding (Bond).

Length of Hair This is where you write in the length of hair you will use. Usual lengths available are: 8", 12", 16", 20" or 24".

Color of Hair Here you will indicate the color of hair you will be ordering. (This is not necessarily the final color. You may be coloring the hair to match your client's hair.)

Cost per inch If you are charging your client by the inch, you will use this column.
(See *Hair Costing Sheet* Figure 6 and *Hair Pricing Sheet* Figure 7).

Width of Track Measure the width of each track and write the inches per track here.

Times Density If you are sewing only one weft on a track, the density will be 1. If you are doing double density, then the density will be 2. (No more than double density is ever recommended. Two wefts sewn onto one track is enough. Any more and you will have matting problems.)

= Total Number of inches Multiply the *density* (1 or 2) by the *width of track* and you will have the total number of inches required for this track.

Price for Hair Now, multiply the *cost per inch* by the *total number of inches* and you will have the price you will charge your client for the hair on this track. Or, some stylists charge the client for the entire weft (or wefts) purchased. (Refer to Figures 6 and 7.)

Estimated Number of Hours Here you will write down the estimated number of hours (or fraction thereof) it will take you to do this track. Another approach for pricing the time required for attachment of the hair extensions is by track. Some stylists use the forumla of two times the price of a haircut per track. In other words if you charge $50.00 for a haircut, you would charge $100.00 per track.

Perm Price per inch You have the option of purchasing factory permed hair or custom perming the hair. (For ideas on how to price permed hair see Figures 6 and 7.) Another approach for pricing for perming the weft is to use your standard prices for permanent wave services.

Totals Totals include: Number of inches; Price for hair; Estimated number of hours and; Perm price per inch.

```
                        PRICING WORK SHEET
┌─────────────────────────────────────────┬─────────────────────────────────────────┐
│ FIRST TIME PRICES                       │ MAINTENANCE PRICES                      │
│ Consultation Fee ............ _____   │                                         │
│ Services to Client's Hair               │ Services to Client's Hair               │
│ Shampoo and Finish .......... _____   │ Shampoo and Finish .......... _____   │
│ Hair Cut and Finish ......... _____   │ Hair Cut and Finish ......... _____   │
│ Intense Conditioning Treatment _____  │ Intense Conditioning Treatment _____  │
│ Permanent, Relaxing, Soft Waves _____ │ Permanent, Relaxing, Soft Waves _____ │
│ products_____      │ products_____      │
│ _____      │ _____      │
│ _____      │ _____      │
│ _____      │ _____      │
│ Color Treatments ............ _____   │ Color Treatments ............ _____   │
│ notes_____      │ notes_____      │
│ _____      │ _____      │
│                                         │                                         │
│ Services for Extensions                 │ Services for Extensions                 │
│ Price for Hair .............. _____   │ Price for Hair .............. _____   │
│ Perming Hair ................ _____   │ Perming Hair ................ _____   │
│ Coloring Hair ............... _____   │ Coloring Hair ............... _____   │
│ notes_____      │ notes_____      │
│ Tracking Est # hrs_____   │ Tracking Est # hrs_____   │
│ Shampoo _____ ...$_____      │ Shampoo _____ ...$_____      │
│ Conditioner _____ ...$_____      │ Conditioner _____ ...$_____      │
│ Conditioner _____ ...$_____      │ Conditioner _____ ...$_____      │
│ Conditioner _____ ...$_____      │ Conditioner _____ ...$_____      │
│ Home-Care Kit ........$_____         │ Home-Care Kit ........$_____         │
│ _____ ...$_____      │ _____ ...$_____      │
│ _____ ...$_____      │ _____ ...$_____      │
│ _____ ...$_____      │ _____ ...$_____      │
│ Sales Tax ............$_____         │ Sales Tax ............$_____         │
│ Price Home Care Items ....... _____   │ Price Home Care Items ....... _____   │
│                                         │                                         │
│ TOTAL AMOUNT DUE ............ _____   │ TOTAL AMOUNT DUE ............ _____   │
│ Less Consultation Fee ....... _____   │ Approximate date for re-do .. _____   │
│ Sub Total ................... _____   │ Notes_____       │
│ Deposit of 50% .............. _____   │                                         │
│ Balance Due ................. _____   │                                         │
├─────────────────────────────────────────┴─────────────────────────────────────────┤
│                    FORMS TO COMPLETE or TO DISCUSS                                │
│   ☐ Chemical Services Release    ☐ Hair Extension Agreement   ☐ Model's Release  │
│   ☐ Hair Extension Release                                    ☐ Home Care Instructions │
└───────────────────────────────────────────────────────────────────────────────────┘
  © Copyright 1990 Garland Drake International ®   Used with permission from Garland Drake International ®   1207/GDIF01
```

Figure 4 – Page 4 of 4

Pricing Work Sheet

Probably the question asked most by stylists is, "How do you price hair extension services?" And by clients, "How much does it cost?" Because of the complexity of hair extension services, there is no easy answer.

There are two sides to the Pricing Work Sheet. The left side is designed to work out First Time Prices whereas the right side is for Maintenance Prices. Using *your Price List you will then work out the price.*

First Time Prices

Consultation Fee is the amount you are charging for this consultation. Stylists will base this fee usually on half of what they would earn during the same period of time. In other words if your time is worth $100.00 per hour, you would charge $50.00 per consultation.

Services to Client's Hair are the charges relative to any services you will be doing to the client's own hair.

Services for Extensions are the charges for services to the hair and your charges for attachment. These include:

    Price for Hair
    Perming Extension Hair
    Color Extension Hair
    Tracking Estimated Number of Hours

Price Home Care Items is the price you will charge for all the home care items you'll list above. You don't give your client the option of what hair care items to take home. You *"prescribe"* them and *include* them in your initial pricing. Sales tax will have to be added to these items. Then you will place the total of these items on this line.

Total Amount Due is a total of all items in the above column.

Less Consultation Fee is the amount of the consultation fee you are going to credit to your client if you will be doing the hair extensions. (If not, your client will owe you for this fee.)

Sub Total You have now subtracted the consultation fee from the total amount due which will equal the Sub Total due.

Deposit of 50% This is one-half (1/2) of the Sub Total amount and will be the amount that you request your client to pay *before* booking their appointment, ordering the hair, etc. If, after you have completed your consultation, your client wants to "think about it" – be sure to *collect the consultation fee*. When the client does decide to have you do the hair extension services, you can then credit this amount to their total due. However, remember, *before* you book the appointment and order the hair – get the deposit amount you have worked out on this pricing work sheet.

Balance Due is the amount your client will owe you after paying the deposit and upon completion of the services.

Maintenance Prices
It is very important to let your client know approximately how much it will cost to maintain the hair extensions. It the client takes proper care of the hair, usually there will be no additional price for hair and for services to the hair. Also, usually the second time you do a client it goes faster. But, remember, you have to un-do the tracking.

I strongly suggest you don't use the term "tightening" when referring to follow-up services for hair extensions. There are some techniques, such as thread weaving and even individual braiding, where the stylist will "tighten" the track by pushing the threads or individual braid up the hair shaft closer to the scalp. However, this is not the best approach to maintaining the hair extension style.

I am a firm believer in re-doing the track/braids after they have grown out because I think you should reposition them. This reduces the stress on the root of specific strands. Also, for sanitation purposes and a healthy scalp, you should cleanse and massage the scalp, which can best be done without the extensions in place. It may only be semantics, only words, but these words bring a vision in your client's mind.

Again, you need to always remember time you spend re-doing a style. You must charge appropriately for that time. Usually the maintenace prices are one-third (1/3) to one-half (1/2) less expensive than the first time prices.

SERVICES PRICE SHEET

SERVICES TO CLIENT'S HAIR	Technicians	Director
Basic Services		
Shampoo and Finish	25.00+	30.00+
"w/Thermal Straightening	35.00+	40.00+
Hair Cut and Finish *	40.00+	50.00+
"w/Thermal Straightening *	50.00+	60.00+
Intense Conditioning Treatment	20.00+	30.00+
Permanent Waves or Chemical Relaxers		
Short hair/not color-treated †	55.00+	60.00+
Short hair/color-treated †	65.00+	70.00+
Medium/not color-treated †	65.00+	70.00+
Medium/color-treated †	75.00+	80.00+
Long hair/not color-treated	100.00+	105.00+
Long hair/color-treated	125.00+	135.00+
Advanced wraps ‡	125.00+	135.00+
Root Permanent Waves		
add $10.00 to above prices		
Partial Permanent Waves		
not color-treated	55.00+	65.00+
color-treated	65.00+	75.00+
Soft Curl Permanents		
Short hair/not color-treated	75.00+	80.00+
Short hair/color-treated	85.00+	90.00+
Medium/not color-treated	85.00+	90.00+
Medium/color-treated	95.00+	100.00+
Long hair/not color-treated	120.00+	125.00+
Long hair/color-treated	135.00+	150.00+
Advanced wraps ‡	135.00+	150.00+
Color Treatments		
Semi-Permanent	35.00+	40.00+
Re-Touch	40.00+	45.00+
Virgin Hair	50.00+	55.00+
Dimensional	75.00+	80.00+
Dimensional Re-Touch	65.00+	70.00+
Double Process Re-Touch	50.00+	55.00+
Double Process Virgin Hair	100.00+	110.00+
Corrective Color ‡	75.00+	80.00+
Cap Highlighting and Frosting		
Short hair	40.00+	50.00+
Medium hair	55.00+	65.00+
Long hair	75.00+	85.00+
Foil Weave or Re-Touch		
Short hair	55.00+	65.00+
Medium hair	70.00+	80.00+
Long hair	100.00+	110.00+
Partial Foil	55.00+	65.00+

HAIR EXTENSION SERVICES	Technicians	Director
Video & Explanation 30 min.	N/C	N/C
Consultation (applied to services)	50.00+	50.00+
Price of Hair	*Hair Pricing Sheet*	
Permanent Waves		
dark colors hair/per inch	1.00+	1.00+
medium colors hair/per inch	1.00+	1.00+
light colors hair/per inch	1.50+	1.50+
lightest colors hair/per inch	2.00+	2.00+
Coloring Extension Hair		
Coloring (regular)	40.00+	45.00+
Foil Weave	‡	‡
Tracking ** price per hour	80.00+	100.00+
Hair Care Items		
Deep Cleansing Shampoo *16 oz*		11.42
Maximum Moisturizing Shampoo *16 oz*		20.57
Maximum Moisturizing Shampoo *8 oz*		10.28
Maximum Moisturizing Conditioner *16 oz*		14.28
Maximum Moisturizing Conditioner *8 oz*		7.14
Stay-In Conditioner *8 oz*		14.28
Protein Pak *1.5 oz*		7.85
Other Items see pricing on packages		

Notes:
* Includes shampoo
† Prices for either perming or relaxing
‡ Consult with director
** Tracking means all attachment techniques:
  Bonding, Micro-Braiding,
  Individual Braiding, Weaving.

Short hair = to bottom of ear
Medium hair = at jawline
Long hair = shoulder length

Other hair addition services available for falls, wigs and replacements.

Call for an appointment
All consultations and services are by appointment only.

Garland Drake TechCENTER
3900 Birch Street #104, Newport Beach, CA 92660
714/250-2970 • Fax 714/250-8530

Figure 5

SAMPLE SERVICES PRICE SHEET

Introduction

You will need to work up your own price list. Figure 5 is only a suggested format. Be sure to add a + sign behind every item. You always need to have flexibility in pricing so that you can add to the "base" price when appropriate.

Services to Client's Hair

You will notice that this is an ala carte price list with two different prices, one for technicians and one for the director. The left side of the form includes all types of services to all types of hair. *(Hair has no sex and no race.)*

Hair Extension Services

Price of Hair
This is one formula you can use to work out the price you'll charge your client for the hair. This usually averages out to be about a 4 times markup. (See Figures 6 and 7)

Permanent Waves
This is a suggested formula if you are *custom perming* the hair for your client. Or, you may want to use your standard perming prices.

Coloring Extension Hair
In this case coloring hair extensions are listed as $40.00+ to $45.00+. However, if the coloring is not extensive, you may want to give this service to your client for "free." But, let them know you are going to give them a *deal*.

Foil Weave
This should be listed as a separate item from coloring because it is much more involved.

Tracking
If you are using more than one type of attachment technique on a client, pricing this service is easiest done by a per hour price. The recommended per hour price is two times your hair cut price. Other stylists like to charge by the number of tracks added to the client's hair.

Remember, when presented this way, the tracking fee includes making the tracks, attaching the hair, cutting the extended hair, cutting-in the client's hair with the extended hair and finishing the style.

Do not undersell yourself. Your advanced education, your hours of practice, your experience and your time have a higher value than anyother service you can provide to your client.

Hair Care Items
Here are the items that you will be listing on the *Consultation Work Sheet* under **Price Home Care Items.**

HAIR COSTING SHEET

#1 Color	#2 Length	#3 Width	#4 Cost Straight	#5 Cost per inch	#6 PRICE per weft	#7 PRICE per inch	#8 Cost w/Curl	#9 Cost per inch	#10 PRICE per weft	#11 PRICE per inch
Stage 0	8" x	108"								
Brownish	12" x	72"								
Black	16" x	54"								
	20" x	43"								
	24" x	36"								
Stage 1	8" x	108"								
Dark	12" x	72"								
Brown	16" x	54"								
	20" x	43"								
	24" x	36"								
Stage 2	8" x	108"								
Reddish	12" x	72"								
Brown	16" x	54"								
	20" x	43"								
	24" x	36"								
Stage 3	8" x	108"								
Brownish	12" x	72"								
Red	16" x	54"								
	20" x	43"								
	24" x	36"								
Stage 8	8" x	108"								
Yellow	12" x	72"								
Orange	16" x	54"								
	20" x	43"								
	24" x	36"								
Stage 9	8" x	108"								
Yellow	12" x	72"								
	16" x	54"								
	20" x	43"								
	24" x	36"								

© Copyright 1990 Garland Drake International ®   Used with permission from Garland Drake International ®   1207/GDIF08

Figure 6

HAIR COSTING SHEET

The *Hair Costing Sheet* is an example of how you can work out pricing either by inches or by weft. You always need to know the width of the weft so you will have enough hair.

#1 Color
This is the color of hair available.

#2 Length
The length of the hair. Longer lengths cost more. (Note: 20" and 24" hair may not be available by 1996. Even now the prices for this length hair are very expensive.)

#3 Width
The width of the weft is important for you to know so you can be sure that you have enough hair.

#4 Cost of Straight
This is your wholesale cost of the hair straight hair (not factory permed). As an example – the cost of an 8" x 108" weft is $20.00.

#5 Cost per Inch
Divide the *cost* (#4) by the *width* of the weft (#3) to get the cost of the hair by inch. If the cost of an 8" x 108" weft is $20.00 then the cost per inch would be $0.1851. This would round out to $0.19 per inch.

#6 Price of Weft
If you decide to take a mark-up on the total cost of the weft, you would take take the *cost* (#4) times the *mark-up* you desire. If the cost of the hair = $20.00 then the price of the weft would be:

   2 times cost = $40.00
   3 times cost = $60.00
   4 times cost = $80.00

#7 Price per Inch
If you decide to take a mark-up on the hair by the amount of inches you will use – then you would multiply the *cost per inch* (#5) by the *mark-up* you desire. Be sure to round-out the figures. If the cost of 8" x 108" weft is $0.19 per inch then the price of the hair would be:

   2 times cost = $0.38 per inch
   3 times cost = $0.57 per inch
   4 times cost = $0.76 per inch

#8 Cost of Pre-Permed Hair
This is your wholesale cost of the hair that has been permed at the factory. As an example – the cost of an 8" x 108" weft is $30.00.

#9 Cost per Inch
Divide the *cost* (#9) by the *width* of the weft (#3) to get the cost of the hair by inch. If the cost of an 8" x 108" pre-permed weft is $30.00 then the cost per inch would be $0.2777. This would round out to $0.28 per inch.

#10 Price of Weft
If you decide to take a mark-up on the total cost of the weft, you would take take the *cost* (#8) times the *mark-up* you desire. If the cost of the hair = $30.00 then the price of the weft would be:

   2 times cost = $60.00
   3 times cost = $90.00
   4 times cost = $120.00

#11 Price per Inch
If you decide to take a mark-up on the hair by the amount of inches you will use, then you would multiply the *cost per inch* (#9) by the *mark-up*

you desire. Be sure to round-out the figures. If the cost of 8" x 108" weft is $0.28 per inch than the price of the hair would be:

2 times cost = $0.56 per inch
3 times cost = $0.84 per inch
4 times cost = $1.12 per inch

HAIR PRICING SHEET

The *Hair Pricing Sheet* is similar to the *Hair Costing Sheet*. The difference is that this sheet lists *only* the retail prices. It is advisable that you keep this form in your client folder, *not* the *Costing Sheet*. You **do not** want your clients to know your costs.

Also, many salon owners consider the hair a retail item. As such, the owner is responsible for the purchase of the hair. In this situation, usually the stylist receives a commission on the hair at the normal commission rate of retail items. (Payment for services done to the client and to the hair are then treated in the usual manner.) Naturally, in this case, only the *Hair Pricing Sheet is made available to the stylist or client.*

HAIR PRICING SHEET

#1 Color	#2 Length	#3 Width	#4 PRICE Straight per weft	#5 PRICE per inch	#6 PRICE w/Curl per weft	#7 PRICE per inch
Stage 0	8" x	108"				
Brownish	12" x	72"				
Black	16" x	54"				
	20" x	43"				
	24" x	36"				
Stage 1	8" x	108"				
Dark	12" x	72"				
Brown	16" x	54"				
	20" x	43"				
	24" x	36"				
Stage 2	8" x	108"				
Reddish	12" x	72"				
Brown	16" x	54"				
	20" x	43"				
	24" x	36"				
Stage 3	8" x	108"				
Brownish	12" x	72"				
Red	16" x	54"				
	20" x	43"				
	24" x	36"				
Stage 8	8" x	108"				
Yellow	12" x	72"				
Orange	16" x	54"				
	20" x	43"				
	24" x	36"				
Stage 9	8" x	108"				
Yellow	12" x	72"				
	16" x	54"				
	20" x	43"				
	24" x	36"				

© Copyright 1990 Garland Drake International ©
Used with permission from Garland Drake International ©
1207/GDIF09

Figure 7

CHEMICAL SERVICES RELEASE STATEMENT

This release is to be used any time you are doing chemical services to someone who already has damaged or stressed hair. Since you will often be doing corrective work, you will be exposed to more people with hair that is or can be damaged.

Also, remember to do *patch tests* and record this information on the *Chemical Services Record* (Figure 12).

Another thing you will need to consider is the possibility of problems occurring as a result of the client's medical condition or medications they are taking. This is important if you are working with clients who need special attention *because of* their medical condition.

CHEMICAL SERVICES RELEASE STATEMENT

Client's Name:_____

Address:_____

City, State, Zip:_____

Home Telephone:(___)_____ Work Telephone:(___)_____

Condition of Hair:_____

Services done by:_____

I fully understand that the services/treatment which I have requested (listed below), while normally harmless to hair, may be harmful to mine.

Check service(s) to be done.
- ☐ Thermal Straightening Finish............................. initial_____
- ☐ Permanent Waving/Chemical Relaxing .... initial_____
- ☐ Color Treatment .... initial_____
- ☐ Hair Extension Attachment .... initial_____

The reason that the above checked service(s) may be harmful to my hair is because of its condition as a result of:

_____

_____

Therefore, I hereby assume all responsibility and risk for any damage that may result, directly or indirectly, from this requested service.

Date:_____

Client's Signature:_____

Stylist's Signature:_____

Manager/Owner's Signature:_____

© Copyright 1990 Garland Drake International® Used with permission from Garland Drake International® 1207/GDIF02

Figure 8

HAIR EXTENSION AGREEMENT

Our Commitment to Our Clients

The below-named stylist has taken graduate courses in hair extension services and is dedicated to the highest standards of the profession of cosmetology. These standards include education and practices in safe and professionally accepted techniques and products for use on a client's scalp and hair.

As to the pricing of hair extension services, the price quoted is the best estimate. It is difficult to always accurately estimate all aspects of hair extension services, supplies needed or time required. If the price quoted is *under* the actual price, the client will be credited with the difference and the balance due will be adjusted accordingly. It is further agreed that if the price quoted is *over* the actual price, there will be no additional charges.

Professional hair extension services require a team effort. Both the stylist and the client must work together in seeing that the client's own hair and scalp are kept in a healthy condition. It is also important that proper care and with recommended products is done by the client at home, at all times. In addition, the success of hair extension services depends on communication between the stylist and client. To be sure that the client understands how to care for and maintain the hair extension, the client will be given a *free check-up appointment*. This appointment must take place within 12 days after the hair extension service is completed.

The Client's Commitment to Us

It is understood that prior to the hair extension services there will be an investment in product and money including the purchase and preparation of the hair to be used to create the style. It is for this reason that all or part of the deposit is *not* refundable.

It is further understood that time (in which other clients could be scheduled) will be *reserved* for doing the hair extension services and because of this, if for any reason the appointment has to be cancelled, it must be done within 48 hours (2 days) prior to the scheduled appointment. Otherwise, there will be *no* refund of the deposit.

It is important for the stylist to check the condition of a client's scalp, hair and added hair. Without proper follow-up a client could unknowingly be doing something that could be hazardous to his or her own hair, scalp or the added hair. For this reason it is agreed to keep the *free check-up appointment*.

SCHEDULING FOR SERVICES

Service	Date	Time	Service	Date	Time
Permanent/Relaxing/Soft Wave			Hair Extension Services		
Coloring Services			Check-Up Appointment		

Summary of Prices
Total Amount Due _____
Less Consultation Fee _____
Sub Total _____
Deposit of 50% _____
Balance Due _____

Method of Payment
☐ Check # _____ ☐ Cash
☐ Card # _____
Exp. Date ___/___

Today's Date _____
Client's Signature: _____
Stylist's Signature _____
Manager/Owner's Signature _____

☐ Client's copy   ☐ File copy

© Copyright 1991 Garland Drake International
Used with permission from Garland Drake International ®
Form/GDIF03

Figure 9

HAIR EXTENSION AGREEMENT

The *Hair Extension Agreement* should be read by your client as a part of your consultation. Although a sample of this form is included, I'd like you to *carefully* read the words of this agreement.

It goes as follows:

Our Commitment to Our Clients

The below-named stylist has taken graduate courses in hair extension services and is dedicated to the highest standards of the profession of cosmetology. These standards include education and practices in safe and professionally-accepted techniques and products for use on a client's scalp and hair.

Relative to the pricing of hair extension services, the price quoted is the best estimate. It is difficult to always accurately estimate all aspects of hair extension services, supplies needed or time required. If the actual price is *less than* the price quoted, the client will be credited with the difference and the balance due, adjusted accordingly, will be less. It is further agreed that if the actual price is *more than* the quoted price, there will be *no additional charges*.

Professional hair extension services require a team effort. Both the stylist and the client must work together to make sure that the client's own hair and scalp are kept in a healthy condition. It is also important that proper care with recommended products is done by the client at home, at all times. In addition, the success of hair extension services depends on communication between the stylist and client. To be sure that the client understands how to care for and maintain the hair extension, the client will be given a free check-up appointment. This appointment must take place within 12 days after the hair extension service was completed.

The Client's Commitment to Us

It is understood that, prior to the hair extension services, there will be an investment in product and money including the purchase and preparation of the hair to be used to create the style. It is for this reason that all or part of the deposit is not refundable.

It is further understood that time (in which other clients could be scheduled) will be reserved for doing the hair extension services and because of this, if for any reason the appointment has to be cancelled, it must be done at least 48 hours (two days) prior to the scheduled appointment. Otherwise, there will be no refund of the deposit.

After the hair extension services, it is important for the stylist to check the condition of a client's scalp, hair and added hair. Without proper follow-up, a client could unknowingly be doing something that could be hazardous to his or her own hair, scalp or the added hair. For this reason the client agrees to keep the *free check-up appointment*.

Scheduling for Services

You will have booked the appropiate appointments, collected the deposit and then complete the information at the bottom portion of the *Hair Extension Agreement,* sign it, have the manager or owner sign it.

This form is to be made in *duplicate*. One copy you will give to your client and one copy you will place in your client's file folder with all the other forms.

MODEL'S AGREEMENT/RELEASE FORM

This form is appropriate if you are going to take before-and-after pictures of your client. Taking pictures of your clients is helpful to build your book. Also, you may be able to submit your pictures for publication. And, *don't forget,* take before and after pictures of the styles you do for your friends, co-workers and family members. You never know, you may need this form. You'll need this form if you are going to publish the pictures in your local newspapers, in trade magazines or anywhere else. So, any time you take a picture, be sure to get a release signed!

MODEL'S AGREEMENT/RELEASE FORM

I hereby give permission to _____
to take pictures of my current hairstyle (the before picture) and of my hairstyle after my extension services (after picture). Further, I agree that _____
may use these photographs, tapes, films, videos and/or interviews in whatever way that _____ feels is proper.

I hereby release all claims on the photographs, tapes, films, videos and/or interviews.

Date: _____

Print Model's Name: _____

Address: _____

City: _____ State: _____ Zip: _____

Phone #: _____

Model's Signature: _____

Stylist: _____

Witnessed: _____

© Copyright 1990 Garland Drake International ®   Used with permission from Garland Drake International ®   1207/GDIF04

Figure 10

HAIR EXTENSION RELEASE

After you have *completed* the *hair extension services,* be sure to have your client sign this release. There are some problems with lawsuits from hair extension clients. I think one of the biggest problems stems from ignorance and jealousy. The reasons given are almost never the real reasons. The motivation more times than not is pressure from a "friend" or spouse. It is so sad that people are often influenced or pressured by people who want to "pull them down." But then, that is nothing new. There is hardly anything, next to plastic surgery, that is so dramatic as hair extension services. As a result, jealousy of others, the need to exert power over another person, are usually the reasons "friends" put pressure on your client. Of course, if you've been in the business for any length of time, you've seen it before. You've created a great style, or colored a client's hair and it looks beautiful and appropriate. The client leaves loving her new look. Lo and behold, a few days later she is back – with some kind of story about why she hates it.

It's much worse with hair extension services. It is best to be prepared for such an event. There is a good chance that by following the suggestions in this chapter you'll be able to avoid such situations.

HAIR EXTENSION SERVICES RELEASE STATEMENT

I agree that I will return for my free check-up. I also agree to use only the products recommended by my stylist.

Date for *free check-up:*_____

I have had a consultation relative to the correct care of my hair extensions and fully understand how to care for my new hair.

I am satisfied with my new hair extension style and therefore, I hereby assume all responsibility for the care of my own hair and the hair extensions.

Date:_____

Client's Signature:_____

Stylist's Signature:_____

Manager/Owner's Signature:_____

© Copyright 1990 Garland Drake International ®
Used with permission from Garland Drake International ®

1290/GD1F05

Figure 11

CHEMICAL SERVICE RECORD

Because hair extension services are special, I recommend that you make a file folder for each client. You can keep all the forms discussed in this chapter in the folder. In addition, you'll need a more elaborate chemical services record form than you usually use. If you are working in a team environment, you particularly need to keep track of prices and who did each particular service.

CHEMICAL SERVICES RECORD

Name: _____ Date: _____
Stylist: _____ Phone #: _____
Hair Form: Previous Product Used _____
Notes _____
Hair Color: _____
Previous Product Used _____
Notes _____
Chemical Curling Test Strand: Date _____ Product _____
Results _____
Notes:

Date	Curling – Product, Rod Size, Type Wrap, Processing Time, Results	Price	by

Hair Coloring Patch Test: Date _____ Product _____
Results _____
Notes:

Date	Coloring – Product, Description, Processing Time, Results	Price	by
Date	Extension Curling – Product, Rod Size, Type Wrap, Processing Time, Results	Price	by
Date	Extension Coloring – Original Color, Product, Notes	Price	by

© Copyright 1990 Garland Drake International ®   Used with permission from Garland Drake International ®   1207/GDIF07

Figure 12

HOME CARE INSTRUCTIONS

Introduction

Never leave your clients on their own when it comes to home care instructions. During your consultation you will have explained what kind of home care they will need to do. Then, during the time you are attaching the hair, you'll have time to give them complete, detailed instructions, including more information about the products you want them to use. After you have completed the style, either you or your assistant should spend another 10 minutes giving them the products they are to use at home. Some stylists include the price of the shampoo and conditioners in their initial price. Others explain what these are and what the prices are. Your hair extension clients will really listen to you as to what products to use because, after all, they have a substantial investment in their hair. You don't want them going to the local drugstore and buying the wrong products. So, for their sake, and for your additional income, be sure to sell them the correct products.

Put It In Writing

The major thing to impress on your clients is to *use common sense* when caring for their hair and hair extensions.

Encourage your clients to ask you a lot of questions. *There is no such thing as a stupid question.*

Figure 13 is a *Home Care Instruction* four page booklet. This is what it says:

Welcome to the world of hair extensions!
When you get home you may then ask yourself "How will I ever be able to wash, dry and style all this hair?" Well, don't wait until you get home. Before you leave the salon you should have *all* your questions answered.

First, for people who have grown their hair long or who have thick hair – they know how to "live" with this hair – it became part of them month by month, over the years. For you, this may be a completely new experience. You may not be used to thick hair and/or long hair.

There is one very basic rule to follow. It is *use common sense* when caring for your hair and hair extensions. Don't pull on them, brush them roughly, let the wind or water tangle and mat them or go too long before visiting your stylist for a check-up.

Follow the guidelines in this booklet and *use common sense*. Your extensions will be what they are meant to be, an "extension" of yourself.

You are special
Remember, not everyone can wear extensions. You need to dedicate time and money for their proper care. But, if you are *willing* to make this commitment – enjoy your new look!

Learning to Love and Live with Your New Hair
Home Care Instructions for your 100% Human Hair Extensions

Welcome to the world of hair extensions!
When you get home you may ask yourself "How will I ever be able to wash, dry and style all this hair?" Well, don't wait until you get home. Before you leave the salon you should have *all* your questions answered.

First, for people who have grown their hair long or who have thick hair – they know how to "live" with this hair – it became part of them month to month, over the years. For you, this may be a completely new experience. You may not be used to thick hair and/or long hair.

There is one very basic rule to follow. It is *use common sense* when caring for your hair and hair extensions. Don't pull on them, brush them roughly, let the wind or water tangle and mat them or go too long before visiting your stylist for a check-up. Follow the guidelines in this booklet and *use common sense.* Your extensions will be what they are meant to be, an "extension" of yourself.

You are special
Remember, not everyone can wear extensions. You need to dedicate time and money for their proper care. But, if you are *willing* to make this commitment – enjoy your new look!

Problems?
Call your stylist **immediately** if you notice any problems or have any questions. Remember to use *only* the products *recommended by your stylist.* Your stylist cannot be responsible for damage caused to your hair, your scalp or the extended hair if you do not follow the instructions in this booklet and do not use the products recommended. It is important to your stylist that you are happy with your extensions!

Moisturizing conditioner: A moisturizing conditioner is as the name implies – a conditioner designed to moisturize the hair. This type of conditioner is applied, generously to wet hair, right after shampooing. It is left on the hair for 5 minutes then rinsed thoroughly.

Intensive conditioner: An intensive conditioner is *required* for hair extensions. Shampoo your hair then apply the intensive conditioner to the wet hair. Carefully work thoroughly into the hair. Depending on the amount of conditioning required you will leave it on the hair for 10 to 30 minutes. Also depending on the requirements you may cover with a plastic bag and/or you may need to go under a hairdryer. After the conditioning treatment is completed, rinse the hair.

Conditioning Procedures
If shampooing daily: After shampooing apply a moisturizing conditioner. Once a week, have an intensive conditioning treatment at the salon or follow your stylist's instructions on proper procedures for a home care treatment.

If shampooing every other day: Moisturizing conditioner after each shampooing and intensive conditioning every two weeks.

If shampooing once a week: Moisturizing conditioner after shampooing and intensive conditioning every two weeks.

Styling Instructions
When using a curling iron – be cautious. Extreme heat can damage the extensions. Because of the length and thickness of the hair, you may not feel the heat you are applying. Too much heat can damage *hair* – including your extensions. Be careful. You can use the *same* styling tools on your hair extensions that you use on your own hair. Since the hair in your extensions has been processed, it may be more delicate than your own hair. Hot rollers, curling irons, regular cone rollers, etc. are all acceptable for use on your extensions. However, beware of any extra heat, particularly at the top of the weft, near your scalp.

Sleeping Instructions
Never go to bed with wet hair! For long hair, it is advisable to braid your hair before sleeping. This keeps the extensions from tangling and matting. Also, sleeping on a satin pillowcase can help keep the hair from getting "roughed up" from the friction caused by other materials.

Combing Instructions
Hold the base of the extensions firmly against your head with one hand while combing them carefully with a wide-tooth comb or wire (wig) brush. Do not force the comb or brush through the extensions. Treat them very gently. Apply stay-in conditioner if possible.

Shampooing Instructions
Before shampooing, spray your hair with a stay-in conditioner. Then remove any and all tangles with a wire (wig) brush or a wide tooth comb.

If your hair extensions are attached with individual braids, use your finger tips to separate the braided hair from your natural hair, then brush with a wire brush.

Wash and rinse your hair *gently!* **Do not rub!** Make sure to cleanse your scalp thoroughly, using *only* a shampoo recommended by your stylist. Regardless of the method used to attach the extensions to your hair, the scalp area needs the most attention. For long hair (16" or longer) braid your extensions into one large braid *before washing your hair. This will help avoid tangles.*

Reasons Your Extensions Need Conditioning
For hair extensions conditioning is *extremely* important! The extended hair **does not receive** your own natural oils from your scalp. To avoid matting and tangling, you will need to condition your extended hair on a regular basis. Other things that you do, or that happen to your hair that also make conditioning important are:
- Loss of moisture due to climate
- Chemical services done to the hair
- Use of styling products containing waxes or alcohol
- Use of blow dryers and/or curling irons
- Long exposure to water (swimming, water-skiing)
- Exposure to heat and water (hot tubs, sauna, steam room)

Conditioning Product Descriptions
There are three kinds of conditioning products you will need to use for the proper care of hair extensions. These are: stay-in, Moisturizing and intensive.

Stay-in conditioner: A stay-in conditioner is designed to allow you to minimize the friction caused when combing or brushing your hair which can ruffle or "snag" your hair's cuticle. This conditioner can and should be used almost anytime you comb or brush your hair whether it is wet or dry. (Naturally, you don't want to use it when finishing a style – mainly when you **are** combing/brushing to detangle your hair.)

Special Situations
After swimming in chlorinated or salt water, using a jacuzzi, or exposing the extensions to other such environments, use stay-in conditioners to help comb out any tangles. Immediately your hair should be shampooed and then given an intensive conditioning treatment. *Never let your hair dry with any tangles in it!*

Hair Re-growth
Everyone is constantly losing old hair and growing new hair. The hair that you normally lose each day will be captured in the tracking (braids or threads) or in the bonding that are the foundation for your extensions. Ordinarily, this "old" hair would be coming out in your comb, brush or when you shampoo. Don't be alarmed if there is some of your own hair attached to the bonding or if hair is loose when your tracks are unbraided. This is natural. However, if you feel the amount of loss is abnormal – be sure to discuss this with your stylist.

Hazardous Situations
You may not be able to wear extensions if you are participating in active water sports such as water skiing, scuba diving and so on. The length of time your extensions are exposed to water, and the type of water (the pH balance of the water) can cause swelling of the cuticle of your own hair and particularly of the extended hair. In addition, the roughness of the activities in which you participate may cause the hair to tangle (as would any long hair). Be sure to discuss this with your stylist.

Your stylist is

© Copyright 1990 Garland Drake International®   Form/GDIF13
Used with permission from Garland Drake International®

Figure 13

Problems?
Call your stylist **immediately** if you notice any problems or have any questions. Remember to use *only* the products *recommended by your stylist*. Your stylist cannot be responsible for damage caused to your hair, your scalp or the extended hair if you do not follow the instructions in this booklet and do not use the products recommended. It is important to your stylist that you are happy with your extensions!

Combing Instructions
Hold the base of the extensions firmly against your head with one hand while combing them carefully with a wide-tooth comb or wire (wig) brush. Do not force the comb or brush through the extensions. Treat them very gently. Apply stay-in conditioner if possible.

Shampooing Instructions
Before shampooing, spray your hair with a stay-in conditioner. Then remove any and all tangles with a wire (wig) brush or a wide tooth comb.

If your hair extensions are attached with individual braids, use your finger tips to separate the braided hair from your natural hair, then brush with a wire brush.

Wash and rinse your hair *gently!* **Do not rub!** Make sure to cleanse your scalp thoroughly, using *only* a shampoo *recommended by your stylist*. Regardless of the method used to attach the extensions to your hair, the scalp area needs the most attention. For long hair (16" or longer) braid your extensions into one large braid *before* washing your hair. This will help avoid tangles.

Reasons Your Extensions Need Conditioning
For hair extensions conditioning is *extremely* important! The extended hair **does not receive** your own natural oils from your scalp. To avoid matting and tangling, you will need to condition your extended hair on a regular basis. Other things that you do, or that happen to your hair that also make conditioning important are:

- Loss of moisture due to climate
- Chemical services done to the hair
- Use of styling products containing waxes or alcohol
- Use of blow dryers and/or curling irons
- Long exposure to water (swimming, water-skiing)
- Exposure to heat and water (hot tubs, sauna, steam room)

Conditioning Product Descriptions
There are three kinds of conditioning products you will need to use for the proper care of hair extensions. These are:

- Stay-in
- Moisturizing
- Intensive

Stay-in conditioner: A stay-in conditioner is designed to allow you to minimize the friction caused when combing or brushing your hair which can ruffle or "snag" your hair's cuticle. This conditioner can and should be used almost anytime you comb or brush your hair whether it is wet or dry. (Naturally, you don't want to use it when finishing a style – mainly when you are combing/brushing to detangle your hair.)

Moisturizing conditioner: A moisturizing conditioner is as the name implies – a conditioner designed to moisturize the hair. This type of conditioner is applied, generously to wet hair, right after shampooing. It is left on the hair for 5 minutes then rinsed thoroughly.

Intensive conditioner: An intensive conditioner is *required* for hair extensions. Shampoo your hair then apply the intensive conditioner to the wet hair. Carefully work thoroughly into the hair. Depending on the amount of conditioning required you will leave it on the hair for 10 to 30 minutes. Also depending on the requirements you may cover with a plastic bag and/or you may need to go under a hairdryer. After the conditioning treatment is completed, rinse the hair.

Conditioning Procedures – If shampooing daily:
After shampooing apply a moisturizing conditioner. Once a week, have an intensive conditioning treatment at the salon or follow your stylist's instructions on proper procedures for a home care treatment.

Conditioning Procedures – If shampooing every other day:
Moisturizing conditioner after each shampooing and intensive conditioning every two weeks.

Conditioning Procedures – If shampooing once a week:
Moisturizing conditioner after shampooing and intensive conditioning every two weeks.

Styling Instructions
When using a curling iron – be cautious. Extreme heat can damage the extensions. Because of the length and thickness of the hair, you may not feel the heat you are applying. Too much heat can damage *hair* – including your extensions. Be careful. You can use the *same* styling tools on your hair extensions that you use on your own hair. Since the hair in your extensions has been processed, it may be more delicate than your own hair. Hot rollers, curling irons, regular cone rollers, etc. are all acceptable for use on your extensions. However, beware of any extra heat, particularly at the top of the weft, near your scalp.

Sleeping Instructions
Never go to bed with wet hair! For long hair, it is advisable to braid your hair before sleeping. This keeps the extensions from tangling and matting. Also, sleeping on a satin pillowcase can help keep the hair from getting "roughed up" from the friction caused by other materials.

Special Situations

After swimming in chlorinated or salt water, using a jacuzzi, or exposing the extensions to other such environments, use stay-in conditioner to help comb out any tangles. Immediately your hair should be shampooed and then given an intensive conditioning treatment. *Never let your hair dry with any tangles in it!*

Hair Re-growth

Everyone is constantly losing old hair and growing new hair. The hair that you normally lose each day will be captured in the tracking (braids or threads) or in the bonding that are the foundation for your extensions. Ordinarily, this "old" hair would be coming out in your comb, brush or when you shampoo. Don't be alarmed if there is some of your own hair attached to the bonding or if hair is loose when your tracks are unbraided. This is natural. However, if you feel the amount of loss is abnormal – be sure to discuss this with your stylist.

Hazardous Situations

You may not be able to wear extensions if you are participating in active water sports such as water skiing, scuba diving and so on. The length of time your extensions are exposed to water, and the type of water (the pH balance of the water) can cause swelling of the cuticle of your own hair and particularly of the extended hair. In addition, the roughness of the activities in which you participate may cause the hair to tangle (as would any long hair). Be sure to discuss this with your stylist.

A Personalized Prescription

You, the stylist, should give your client a *personalized prescription* for products to use at home.

Shampoo

When discussing the client's home care habits *(Consultation Work Sheet Figure 1)* you need to determine if you feel that the client is shampooing their hair too often or too seldom. Daily shampooing is OK for hair extension clients but they must be willing to do the extra maintenance required. However, if the client does not shampoo at least weekly you will need to impress this client with the need for healthy habits. You may even want to consider a *special salon maintenance program* for this client. That is, you may want to offer this client a weekly shampoo and style deal like an insurance policy. They could pay you each month a flat fee for four appointments per month.

Under the category of shampoo, also remember any color enhancing product the client may need – such as a temporary rinse or a color refresher shampoo.

For the clients who will be shampooing their own hair at home, be sure to provide (sell) them the correct shampoo for the proper maintenence of the hair extensions. Make sure they will have enough product to last until their next scheduled appointment.

Conditioning

Your clients will require at least two conditioners. First, they need a stay-in conditioner. Second, they need a moisturizing conditioner.

If the clients are not weekly customers, they will need an intensive conditioner.

You must impress your clients with the importance of conditioning! This is a must for the proper home care of hair extensions. Be sure they have enough product. Be sure to tell them how much and how often they should use each product.

Styling Products

Don't leave your clients floundering around when it comes to any liquid or electrical styling tools they may need. You should also be their source for styling gels, waxes and/or mousses. Remember, if their color will need refreshing, color styling mousse is an excellent product to provide (sell) your clients.

Brushes, combs, picks are items everyone needs. Be helpful, save your clients the inconvenience of having to go all over town to get the right tools. Everyone needs these items for at home and at work. You are truly serving your clients when you help to provide them with these needed items.

What about a curling iron or a blow-dryer or attachments for the dryer such as a diffuser? Your clients will be so excited about their new hair they won't even think of these details. That is part of your job. Don't assume anything. It's not being "pushy", it's being helpful They may have the items they need now – but because you mentioned these items to them, the next time they need any hair care items they will come to you – their professional hair care consultant.

SUMMARY

There are three assets that contribute to the success of a stylist: good work habits, positive self-image and excellent communication skills.

The initial consultation with a prospective client fulfills several objectives. By assessing such factors as the client's hair condition, facial structure, life style, etc., the stylist is able to determine the best hairstyle and most appropriate technique for that particular client, and then to communicate those ideas clearly.

Proper pricing of goods and services is an important part of the business. The stylist must take into account all the time required to service a client, from consultation through finished style and charge accordingly.

Chapter 9

CASE STUDIES

INTRODUCTION

Real People – Real Hair

In this section, I'd like to share with you a little about some real situations and real clients. I tried to select clients as models who would tell the story, who would be like clients you can expect to have. The clients and stylists who participated in this shoot were fantastic! So that there would be many different kinds of examples, we did seventeen models in only three days, from start to finish!

Nothing was "dummied up." We didn't make the models look bad for their before pictures. We asked them to do their hair just as they would normally do – the best they could. We even had a makeup artist.

The amazing changes you see here are exactly what happens to clients. You'll notice not only a change in their hair – but an overall change – a spark, an attitude that seems to make them glow. In this case, you really can say that the camera doesn't lie.

Attachment Techniques Used

As you will notice, micro filler fiber braiding was done as the tracking method with the wefts sewn on the tracks for fourteen of the models. By the way, among ourselves we call it braid and sew (B & S) but to clients, use the full name often (micro filler fiber braiding) so the client will better appreciate the skills and techniques required.

On two models, we attached the wefts using adhesive bonding and on only one model we used the individual braiding technique.

This style can also be created by using the bonding or individual braiding techniques. Bonding may not stay. The decision as to which technique to use would depend on all the factors discussed earlier in this book: client's hair; life style; desired look; time and money considerations. Will bonding work for this client? It's faster, as a result less expensive, however, not necessarily as long lasting as micro filler fiber braiding or individual braiding. For individual braiding attachment, do you, the stylist, have time to commit? Will the client want to invest the required time and money for this attachment technique and its maintenance?

All these factors you need to consider. After your initial service to a client, you can try different techniques and see what works best.

The Stylists

I invited four of my favorite hair extension stylists to work this shoot. As you look through the following pages, you will observe the number of hours required for each style. These were long days for everyone.

We did all the before pictures on Saturday, then began working on our models' own hair, also on Saturday. The extension services began early Sunday morning. The shoot started Sunday afternoon and we were done at 7:00 pm on Monday. Truly a marathon of styling!

Lee Anthony
At the time of this shoot, Lee lived in Philadelphia, Pennsylvania and worked for Michael Christopher. The month after this photo shoot, he moved to Newport Beach, California and became the Technical and Artistic Director of Garland Drake International. Lee is also a Zotos Creative Designer and Master Educator. The models done by Lee were:

- Wanda
- Ramin
- Janice
- Lynn
- Kathleen
- Erin

James Cristopher Chan
Owns a salon is Las Vegas, Nevada and also is a Zotos Creative Designer and Master Educator. The models done by James were:

- Zettoria
- Candida
- Susan

Douglas Kovalcik
Works in Denver, Colorado and also is a Zotos Creative Designer. This is the second shoot Doug and I have worked on together. The models done by Doug were:

- Arlene
- Marla
- Jennifer
- Alondra

CASE STUDIES

Keiko Shino
From the Newport Beach area of California and a long-time friend. She has worked with me for many years helping to develop hair extension techniques. The models done by Keiko were:

Monnique
Dana
Leann
Larry

The Creative Team

Of course, everything was a team effort, everyone working with everyone else. Lee Anthony did all the consultations, using the forms shown in Chapter 8, and was the overall director and creative director for this shoot. This was an important aspect because I wanted to make sure that there was a variety of examples for you to see.

Another member of the team was the makeup artist, Denise Landau.

The photographer makes it possible to share the work with you. Everyone involved in this shoot will tell you that Chuck Montague, our photographer, was an exciting and wonderful person to work with. Since our models were "real people" and not used to modeling, having personable photographer was a great help to all of us! Thank you, Chuck!

Clients in Order of Appearance

Monnique – 214
Dana – 216
Leann – 218
Larry – 220
Wanda – 222
Zettoria – 224
Arlene – 226
Marla – 228
Ramin – 230
Jennifer – 232
Alondra – 234
Candida – 236
Janice – 238
Susan – 240
Lynn – 242
Kathleen – 244
Erin – 246

MONNIQUE – Stylist: Keiko Shino

Background Information and Services to Monnique's Hair

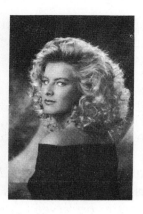

Monnique is 18 years old and works as a secretary for a financial company. She wanted hair extensions for volume and length. She has a petite stature and washes her hair daily.

Her hair had been so heavily foiled that she looked like a double processed blonde. As a result of previous chemical services and improper home care, Monnique's hair was dry, with poor elasticity and very high porosity. Further complicating stylability, her haircut was highly texturized with scissors, which gave it stringy, thin ends.

To correct her hair color, we did a heavy foil weave retouch using 20 volume peroxide and powder bleach to create a golden blonde color. Her hair was then conditioned and lightly trimmed to even out the ends.

Services to Wefts

We decided to custom perm the wefts with an acid perm. White perm rods were used in a spiral wrap pattern. Factory permed wefts called loose curl (white perm rods, 7/16") could have been used.

Since Monnique's hair had quite a bit of gold, we used 12" and 16", stage 8 (yellow-orange) wefts.

Next, the wefts were lowlighted to match her hair color.

Placement Pattern, etc.

With hair as damaged, fine and thin as hers, the micro filler fiber braid (Braid & Sew) was the technique we used.

Two tracks were done to create this style. Track #1 was 8" wide. Two wefts of 16" length hair (double density) were attached. Track #2 was 12" wide. On the bottom of the track (B) 12" length hair was attached whereas on the top (A) 16" hair was used.

Time required for attachment – approximately 2 hours.

Finish/Styling

After razor and scissor cutting, Monnique's style was blown dry and curled with a curling iron.

Optional Approaches

This style can also be created by using the bonding or individual braiding techniques. Bonding may be a problem because of the client's home

CASE STUDIES

care habits. If this style had been done using the individual braiding technique the attachment time would have been approximately 6 to 8 hours.

Comments

When you have a client who has a problem caused by both bad home care habits and improper services/techniques by another stylist, you will need to use a very positive, yet informative approach to this client.

As an example, you *don't* want to say something like, "Boy, did that stylist really mess up your hair! It's over-bleached and that hair cut just ruined it." No, no – *NEVER* put down another stylist's work. If we are to be treated as professionals, we have to act like professionals.

A client with a really bad hair cut usually knows it. The client often is coming to you, the expert, because of this kind of problem. Don't join in with the client in belittling the other stylist. Avoid discussing other's work and concentrate on what YOU can do for the client. Give the client your full professional advice throughout the consultation on all aspects covered on the *Consultation Work Sheet*.

PLACEMENT PATTERN WORK SHEET for MONNIQUE

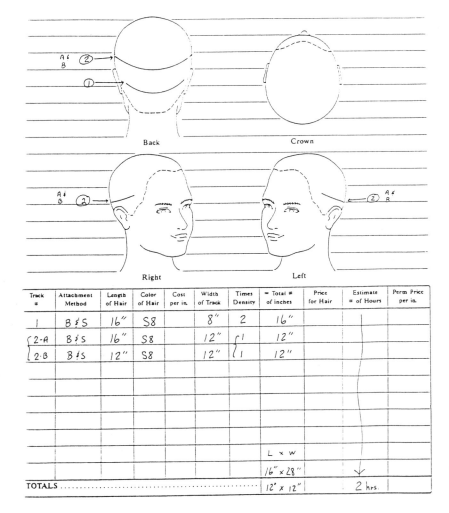

Track #	Attachment Method	Length of Hair	Color of Hair	Cost per in.	Width of Track	Times Density	= Total # of inches	Price for Hair	Estimate = of Hours	Perm Price per in.
1	B & S	16"	S8		8"	2	16"			
2-A	B & S	16"	S8		12"	1	12"			
2-B	B & S	12"	S8		12"	1	12"			
								L × W		
								16" × 28"		
TOTALS								12" × 12"	2 hrs.	

DANA – stylist: Keiko Shino

Background Information and Services to Dana's Hair

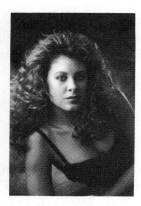

Dana is 18 years old and has just begun her career as a model and actress. The perm is growing out of her hair, which is of a medium-to-fine texture. Several months ago she had some highlights done. Because of chemical services her hair is porous. Also, it is both dry and oily – dry ends, oily scalp. The hair in her temple area recedes slightly. She wanted hair extensions for length and volume.

First, we retouched the highlighting to her hair by foil-weaving her new growth only, using a 9 level gold base color with 20 volume peroxide. Her hair was shampooed and conditioned.

Services to Wefts

Factory permed wefts (with loose curl) could have been used. However, again we custom permed the wefts, using an acid perm with a spiral wrap on white (7/16") rods. In our pre-perm analysis on the weft we determined that it was "strong" enough to test the possibility of using a tint formula perm instead of a bleach formula perm. Our test curl proved this to be true.

The 12" and 16" stage 8 (yellow orange) wefts were next colored to match Dana's own hair by foil weaving. To deposit color on the wefts, we used a level 4 color with 10 volume peroxide.

Placement Pattern, etc.

Three micro filler fiber braids were done to create Dana's style. The 16" wefts on tracks #1 and #2 were sewn on in double density (2 wefts per track). On track #3, the 12" hair was also double density.

The total amount of hair used was – 40" of 16" hair and 20" of 12" hair. The time required for attachment was approximately 3 hours.

Finish/Styling

Razor and scissor cutting was done to give Dana's overall style a finished, natural look. Then her hair was dried with a blow dryer with a diffuser attachment and touched up with a curling iron.

Optional Approaches

This style could have been created by either bonding or individual braids. Because you cannot do double density when bonding, the placement pattern for bonding would have been 6 tracks instead of 3.

CASE STUDIES

If this style had been done by the individual braiding technique, it would have taken 8-10 hours. If this style had been done by the bonding technique, the attachment time would have been approximately 45 minutes.

Comments

Clients, men and women, who are actors or models are excellent clients for hair extensions. Their public image, the physical appearance is very important to their work. They must know how to style their hair and to change the style depending on what "look" is required of them for the occasion. As a result, you need to pay special attention to the area around the hairline to be sure that the wefts cannot be seen.

PLACEMENT PATTERN WORK SHEET for DANA

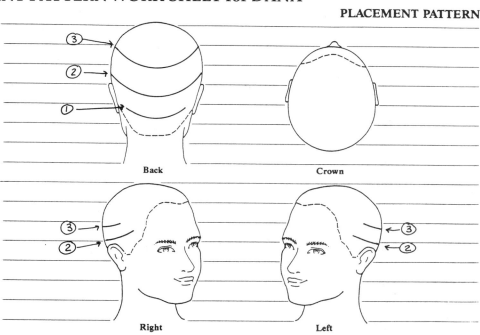

Track #	Attachment Method	Length of Hair	Color of Hair	Cost per in.	Width of Track	Times Density	= Total # of inches	Price for Hair	Estimate # of Hours	Perm Price per in.
1	B&S	16"	S8		8"	2	16"			
2	B&S	16"	S8		12"	2	24"			
3	B&S	12"	S8		10"	2	20"			
							L x W			
							16" x 40"			
TOTALS							12" x 20"		3 hrs	

LEANN – stylist: Keiko Shino

Background Information and Services to Leann's Hair

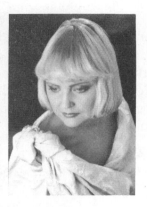

Because Leann has been wearing hair extensions for almost two years her own hair is longer and healthier than it has ever been in her entire life! However, it still is very, very fine and impossible to perm or style. Leann is a communications and PR consultant for several major companies in the beauty industry. In addition to a busy working schedule, Leann was in the last months of her pregnancy. She wanted to continue to wear her hair extensions, but, she also needed to simplify her life as much as possible during this time. So a different placement pattern was created for Leann this time.

Leann's hair was foil-weaved, highlighting the front and the back, in the regrowth area only. Since Leann will have full coverage, it doesn't really matter what color blonde she will be. The objective is to create natural-looking color blends so that if the added hair separates, any hair underneath that might be exposed will blend in and not be detected.

Services to Wefts

Straight texture wefts were used (no perming required) Stage 9 (yellow) wefts were selected. They were shampooed, then decolorized to a lighter shade by doing a "bleach wash." This was done by mixing 20 volume peroxide with powder bleach to a very soupy consistency. The wefts were put in a large plastic mixing bowl with the soupy mixture. They were thoroughly immersed and checked every 2 minutes. The total processing time was 10 minutes. After lightening, the wefts were then shampooed again and conditioned.

Placement Pattern, etc.

The placement pattern was a circular track running clockwise on the top and crown area of Leann's head. A total of 72" of 12" hair was used. The time required for attachment was approximately 4 hours.

Finish/Styling

The added hair was razor and scissor cut into a simple bob style. The style was finished with a curling iron. By the way, shortly after this picture was taken, Leann had a nine-pound baby boy. To her amusement, the comments from the nurses and others were such things as ... "It's wonderful, your son has thick nice hair like you." Only her hairdresser and her husband know.

CASE STUDIES

Optional Approaches

This style cannot be done as successfully with either the individual braiding or the bonding techniques. Only the micro filler fiber braiding technique is appropriate for this style and for Leann's personal comfort.

Comments

Client's with baby-fine hair are perfect candidates for hair extensions. These clients *really want* thick, beautiful hair and never can have it. But, you help them fool mother nature. Also remember, as in Leann's case, client's life style and personal needs are important to consider when doing hair extension services. With the three attachment techniques you have learned – you can accomplish almost anything your client needs. *Just use your imagination!*

PLACEMENT PATTERN WORK SHEET for LEANN

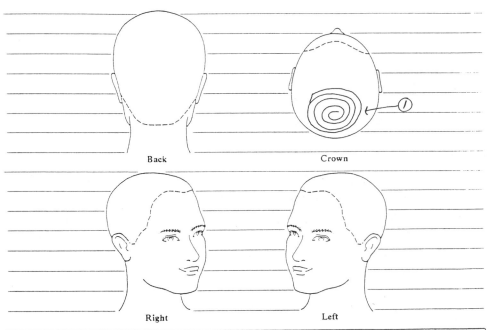

Track #	Attachment Method	Length of Hair	Color of Hair	Cost per in.	Width of Track	Times Density	= Total # of inches	Price for Hair	Estimate # of Hours	Perm Price per in.
1	B & S	12"	59		72	1	72			
						L x W				
TOTALS							12" x 72"		4 hrs.	

LARRY – stylist: Keiko Shino

Background Information and Services to Larry's Hair

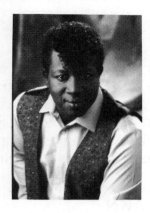

Larry handles deliveries for a major furniture store and in the evenings enjoys his passion for dancing. As a matter of fact, Larry supplements his income with winnings from dancing contests – he's that good. He wanted some hair he could "toss" when dancing. He wanted a fun look.

Larry's hair was very, very short. Because it was so short, any type of attachment technique would be very difficult, if not impossible. So the first step was to restructure his curl, using alternating 3/8" and 5/16" perm rods (gray and pink). After his curl was relaxed his hair was longer – a more workable length.

Services to Wefts

The wefts selected (the non lightened brownish-black color) matched Larry's own hair, so the only service required was to perm the hair. An alkaline perm was used. Yellow flexible perm rods (3/8") were used in a spiral wrap to create a tight curl which his restructured curl.

Placement Pattern, etc.

About 14" of 8" length hair, in the 4 row placement pattern shown in Figure 4, was attached using the individual braid technique. In this situation, individual braid attachment is the best technique to use. The time required to do the attachment was approximately 3 hours.

Finish/Styling

Razor and scissor cutting was done to finish the style.

Optional Approaches

Individual braiding technique is the best method to use for extremely curly and short hair.

In addition, for a client with a physically active life (dancing and moving furniture) there is the possibility that if you used the micro filler fiber braids – the tracks could be an area where perspiration would collect and could cause irritation to the client's scalp.

Another reason for using the individual braiding technique for this style is the style itself. This is the best way to hide the attachment when adding hair in the front hairline.

CASE STUDIES

Comments

Remember, hair has no sex – has no race. As a professional you should be able to service all types of hair – all kinds of clients. Keep up your skills. Learn new and more skills. Attend as many conferences, trade shows and classes as you can.

You are in the *practice* of Cosmetology, just like any other profession. If you treat your work as a JOB – and go into the "shop" each day to do your JOB, probably hair extension services are not for you. But, if you treat your work as a career, a profession, you *know* you must continue to learn.

PLACEMENT PATTERN WORK SHEET for LARRY

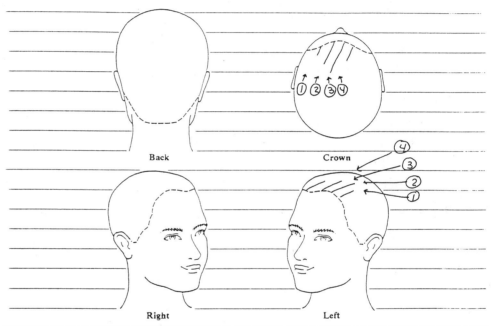

Track #	Attachment Method	Length of Hair	Color of Hair	Cost per in.	Width of Track	Times Density	= Total # of inches	Price for Hair	Estimate # of Hours	Perm Price per in.
1	IB	8"	SO		2"		5-Braids			
2	IB	8"	SO		4"		10-Braids			
3	IB	8"	SO		5"		12-Braids			
4	IB	8"	SO		3"		8-Braids			
TOTALS							L × W 8" × 14"		3 hrs	

WANDA – stylist: Lee Anthony

Background Information and Services to Wanda's Hair

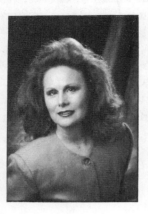

Wanda has a busy life style and has been wearing hair extensions for almost two years. She is in her mid-forties with hair that is not as thick as it used to be. She needs fullness created throughout her hair. Since she likes to wear her hair very long, with the fineness of her hair, the longer it gets the more sparse it appears. You can see through the style.

The only services required were shampooing and conditioning.

Services to Wefts

The wefts were permed, using 9/16" (purple) rods in a spiral wrap. Stage 3 (brownish red) wefts were selected. After perming, they were colored to match her hair.

Placement Pattern, etc.

There were 8 tracks of 12" and 8" hair bonded to Wanda's hair. The total amount of hair (width of wefts) used was 48". Attachment time was approximately 1 hour.

Finish/Styling

To create the finished look, the wefts were razor cut and the style was trimmed. Her hair was dried and set with electric rollers. Brushing and a little back combing in the top area interlocked the wefts with her own hair. This added volume means that instead of having to set her hair daily and doing heavy back-combing to keep the style throughout the day, Wanda sets her hair (on electric rollers) weekly and the style lasts for the entire week!

Optional Approaches

This style can also be created using the braid and sew or individual braiding techniques. However, both of these techniques are more time-consuming, thus more expensive.

For this client, the bonding technique is probably the best method to use. The reasons I say this are because, first, the hair stays bonded to her hair successfully for as long as it should. By this I mean that the wefts stay in place until hair has grown out to a point where they should be removed. Second, the bonding technique is faster, which is a consideration for a person with a busy schedule. And third, it is financially better for her.

Comments

The weekly client, the over 35 client – they are excellent prospects for hair extension services. Do you have clients who come in for a combout during the week, in between their weekly service? Do you have clients whose hair requires more back-brushing that you'd really like to do – but have to just to give them the fullness they want or need?

Bonding in hair for volume may be the biggest part of your hair extension service business! You have clients right now who are perfect prospects.

PLACEMENT PATTERN WORK SHEET for WANDA

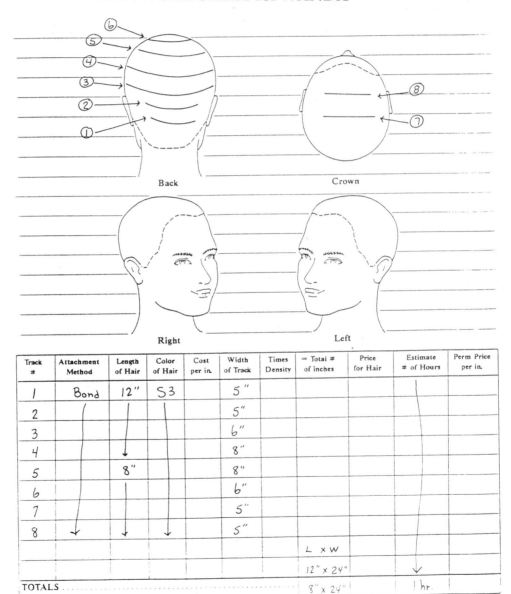

Track #	Attachment Method	Length of Hair	Color of Hair	Cost per in.	Width of Track	Times Density	= Total # of inches	Price for Hair	Estimate # of Hours	Perm Price per in.
1	Bond	12"	S3		5"					
2					5"					
3					6"					
4		↓			8"					
5		8"			8"					
6					6"					
7					5"					
8	↓	↓	↓		5"				↓	
							L × W			
							12" × 24"		↓	
TOTALS							8" × 24"		1 hr.	

ZETTORIA – stylist: James Cristopher Chan

Background Information and Services to Zettoria's Hair

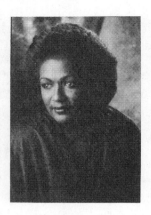

Zettoria works for the US Post Office. Her hair is extremely curly. She relaxes and colors her own hair. Usually she wears hair extensions but removed them for the before picture. Her previous style was thick and long. I had to encourage her to go along with us for this style. Like most people who can't grow long hair, when they *can* have long hair they want it. Really – I mean really – long! Zettoria has a beautiful face, a short neck and a full body. I was exceptionally pleased with the glamorous, professional look of this style. Truly, no one would know she is wearing hair extensions! However, in real life, there are many people like Zettoria who will insist on an inappropriate hairstyle. But you know how that goes. You'll probably have to do a lot of styles that you feel may be too full or too long for the client's facial and/or body features. Just be sure that you are covered in your consultation for any hair care problems the client may face and may decide to blame on you.

The only services required for Zettoria's hair was to shampoo and condition it.

Services to Wefts

Stage 3 (brownish red) wefts matched the color Zettoria used on her own hair without any additional color work to the wefts. They were then permed with 9/16" (purple) rods to create the soft curl look.

Placement Pattern, etc.

There were 3 tracks of 8" hair added to Zettoria's hair. Tracks #1 and #2 were sewn in double density. Track #3 was single density. The total amount of hair used (width of weft) was 42". Attachment time required was approximately 3 hours.

Finish/Styling

The added hair was razor cut and then all the hair was scissor cut to create the finished style.

Optional Approaches

This style could also be created using the individual braid or bonding technique. However, neither of these techniques was advisable for Zettoria. Bonding would not hold on Zettoria's hair because of the hair care products she uses, which contain oils that would break down the bond. Also, Zettoria will probably want to go back to wearing longer hair, and

CASE STUDIES

bonding longer hair is more stressful to the client's own hair. The individual braiding technique for her probably would not be practical nor advisable – particularly if she continues to do her own chemical services at home.

Comments

There is often a conflict between trying to please your client and doing what you feel is best for your client. Zettoria was a good sport about being in this book. This is not her style, nor the way she perceives herself. When I first interviewed her, she was wearing hair extensions in a long, full style. For this book, I could see her as on attractive *professional* woman.

Zettoria is like some customers you will have who will want styles that are not appropriate for the shape of their face, height and/or any of the other physical considerations. It is your job to encourage your client to have appropriate styles. But, if the client really wants another look, you will need to accommodate. This does not mean that "the customer is always right." It means that, as a professional, you are willing to accommodate your customers. Of course, we are only talking about style preference. Taking risks that involve hazards to the client's scalp and/or hair are another issue entirely! And on this, you should not compromise.

PLACEMENT PATTERN WORK SHEET for ZETTORIA

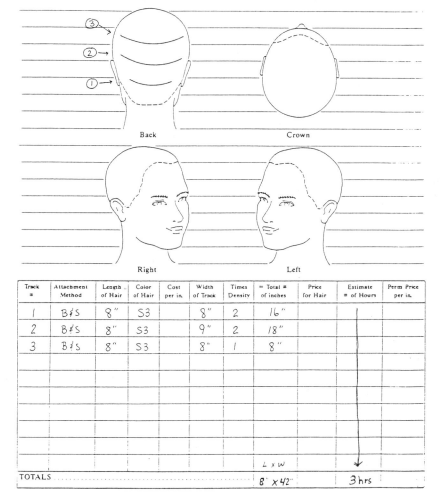

Track #	Attachment Method	Length of Hair	Color of Hair	Cost per in.	Width of Track	Times Density	= Total = of inches	Price for Hair	Estimate # of Hours	Perm Price per in.
1	B&S	8"	S3		8"	2	16"			
2	B&S	8"	S3		9"	2	18"			
3	B&S	8"	S3		8"	1	8"			
								L x W	↓	
TOTALS								8" x 42"	3 hrs	

ARLENE – stylist: Douglas Kovalcik

Background Information and Services to Arlene's Hair

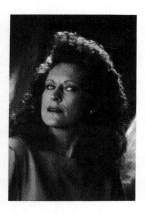

Probably the people who can benefit most from hair extensions are women with baby-fine hair. You know the kind of hair – you try to perm it to give it body, color it to give it life – but nothing really works. Arlene is in her mid-forties and certainly lives a busy life in that she is a mother of two and a Doctor of Chiropractic in private practice. Arlene voiced what I've suspected others have felt. She said, "My hair is something that I inherited, and I thought that it never bothered me. I've lived with it all these years. Now, I can't believe that I'm actually living out one of my chilhood fantasies – which I guess I've suppressed. Wow, I remember dreaming about having full, thick, beautiful hair. But, now that it's a reality – that I have this hair – I can't believe these feelings!"

When we asked Arlene why she wanted to have hair extensions she said, "I want to look sexy!"

One of the reasons Arlene can't grow hair is that her stylist has been giving her perms on top of perms, which naturally causes the hair to break. We did a root perm on the top and sides of her head. I'd like to mention here that many stylists either don't know how to, or are too lazy to, do root perms instead of perm-on-perm. Naturally, as an expert in hair extension services, you will be an expert in the total care of hair – so you will do a root perm whenever required.

In addition to the permanent wave, a semi-permanent color was applied to Arlene's hair.

Services to Wefts

The weft used, a stage 3 (brownish red), was permed to match the curl pattern of Arlene's hair. Also, a semi-permanent color was used to blend her hair and the weft.

Placement Pattern, etc.

There were 3 micro filler fiber braded tracks made as seen on the placement pattern diagram. Tracks #1 and #2 were sewn with double density 12" wefts. Track #3 was done single density with 8" hair. The total amount of hair (width of wefts) used was 52". The approximate attachment time was 3 hours.

Finish/Styling

Arlene's finished look was done by diffused drying and then using a curling iron to give the hair style a little softness.

Optional Approaches

This style could have been created using the bonding or the individual braiding technique. However, because Arlene lives such a busy life, the time required for individual braiding attachment may be a problem. Bonding would be a good option, but remember, you can never be sure how long it will last. For someone as busy are Arlene, if the wefts began to slip, she very likely wouldn't have time to come in immediately to be re-bonded.

Comments

Women who are self employed, especially professional women, are excellent clients for hair extension services – IF – they can be accommodated schedule-wise. Professional women often are "super women" and have very little time for themselves or for "frivolous" things. That is, many professional women that I know, particularily doctors and lawyers, have had to spend so much of their life working and studying, they have had very little interest or experience in "dealing" with their personal appearance, particularly with their hair. However, these women *deserve* the care, expertise and attention of another professional – you.

PLACEMENT PATTERN WORK SHEET for ARLENE

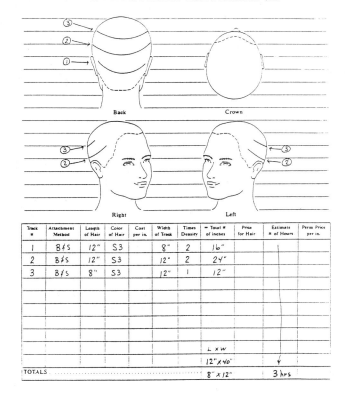

Track #	Attachment Method	Length of Hair	Color of Hair	Cost per in.	Width of Track	Times Density	= Total # of inches	Price for Hair	Estimate # of Hours	Perm Price per in.
1	B&S	12"	S3		8"	2	16"			
2	B&S	12"	S3		12"	2	24"			
3	B&S	8"	S3		12"	1	12"			
							L x W			
							12" x 40"			
TOTALS							8" x 12"		3 hrs	

MARLA – stylist: Douglas Kovalcik

Background Information and Services to Marla's Hair

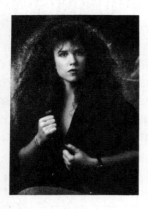

Can you believe that this beautiful young woman is a police dispatcher, goes to college, and skates with a professional roller skating team? Known as Blaze in one of her lives, Marla's life style needs are, naturally, involved. She has a busy life, yet needs to have glamorous, flashy hair.

Again, abuse to the hair is one of the reasons hair extensions are here to stay. We want it all and in this desire often we have too many perms, color too often, or try too many different things on our hair.

We did intensive conditioning to Marla's hair and colored it. This was difficult since she had so many layers-on-layers of many different kinds of color products.

Services to Wefts

Stage 2 (reddish brown) wefts were permed and colored with a semi-permanent red color. The reason we used a semi-permanent color is that we plan on working with Marla over the next few months to help get her hair back to a healthy state. In its current condition it is impossible to achieve the color she desires.

Placement Pattern, etc.

On the track #1, we used 16" hair, double density. Track #2 was done with 16" on the bottom and 12" on the top (double density). Track #3 was done with 12" on the bottom and 8" on the top of the braid. Track #4 was done with 8" hair, single density. This style was created using the micro filler fiber braiding technique. The total amount of hair used (width of the wefts) was 74". The time required for attachment was 3 hours.

Finish/Styling

Marla's finished look was created by razor cutting the hair on the weft, then scissor cutting the total style. Her hair had been diffuser-dried to create a massive, curly, "lion" look.

The second style was created simply by pulling her hair to one side. Since the extensions cannot be seen, you can create many different styles.

Optional Approaches

Because of the amount and length of hair being added, and because of Marla's life style, the bonding technique would not be advisable.

CASE STUDIES

However, this style could also be done using the individual braiding technique. The time required to do individual braiding would be about 10 to 13 hours.

Comments

Marla is the kind of hair extension client you love to have. She needs and wants extensions for fun, for fashion and for her career needs. She is also the type of person willing and delighted to allow the stylist to be the creator. She will follow home care instructions to the letter.

There are many younger women, women who are able to go for it all! The "fight" in the "man's" world is not as difficult for them as it was for their older sisters. Life for them means work and *fun* and *fashion*.

PLACEMENT PATTERN WORK SHEET for MARLA

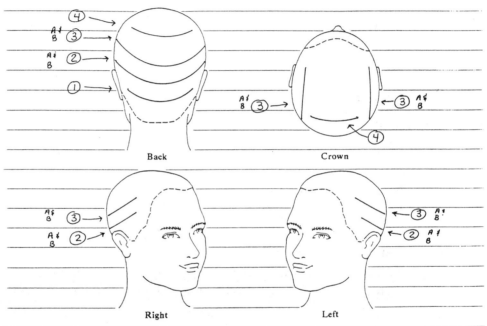

Track #	Attachment Method	Length of Hair	Color of Hair	Cost per in.	Width of Track	Times Density	= Total # of inches	Price for Hair	Estimate # of Hours	Perm Price per in.
1	B & S	16"	S2		8"	2	16"			
2-A		16"			12"	1	12"			
2-B		12"			12"	1	12"			
3-A		12"			13"	1	13"			
3-B		8"			13"	1	13"			
4		8"			8"	1	8"			
							L x W			
							16" x 28"			
							12" x 25"			
TOTALS							8" x 21"		3½ hrs.	

RAMIN – stylist: Lee Anthony

Background Information and Services to Ramin's Hair

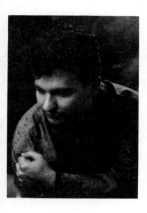

Ramin, training to become an airline pilot, is only 24 years old, and like all the men in his family, his hair is beginning to thin in front and on top. He is not ready for a hair replacement; hair growth preparations have been no help; so hair extensions will add the missing hair to fill out his style.

His hair, in addition to being thin, is very short. Ramin has now grown his own hair longer, making attachment easier.

Only a deep cleansing shampoo was required for Ramin's own hair.

Services to Wefts

The natural brownish-black color of Chinese or Indian hair was a perfect match for Ramin's own hair. No color work was required.

To create the desired texture, the weft was permed with alkaline perm using 3/8" rods (gray).

Placement Pattern, etc.

Ramin was not sure what hair extensions would be like, if he would be able to care for them or if he really wanted to do this. So we decided to use the bonding technique so he could try it out without too much investment. The style was created by first adding hair in the front, dealing with the most difficult area that needed coverage (tracks #1, #2 and #3). Track #4 is where the "split" had to be camouflaged to help achieve the natural hair direction look. Then tracks #5 through #7 were added to complete the coverage. The time required for attachment was 1 hour.

Finish/Styling

The hair dried naturally. The curl formation covered the thin area of Ramin's front and camouflaged the attachment.

Optional Approaches

For a longer-lasting style, it can be created with the individual braiding technique. As a matter-of-fact, several months later, we did do individual braids. That attachment technique was much more practical for Ramin to manage and was not detectable.

Comments

When we read the story of Sampson and Delilah – the point of the story involves human weaknesses and betrayal. But, I've wondered if there is not some reading-between-the-lines there. Many men who are losing their hair are very concerned about it. Are they losing their strength? But then, since more men have hair loss problems than women and men have less options in solving this problem, it is natural that they would be concerned about it.

In 1977 I wrote a booklet about men's hair replacements and was very involved in developing the product, sales and marketing of replacements. However, for several reasons I did not stay in that part of the business. One of the reasons had to do with the education and distribution channels available in those years. I have always believed that adding hair belongs to the licensed cosmetologist/barber industry. It's taken a few years – but finally – here we are. This book is designed to teach you only three of the most important attachment techniques for hair extensions. This is the beginning.

For clients like Ramin, and you see many clients like him in the early stages of balding you can use your knowledge of hair extensions to give them the hair they need now. This kind of client never needs to "go bald" and then make the big jump to a hair replacement. You start with changing the style to help you add hair where it's needed and still be able to hide the attachment technique. But be ready – it won't be long before you need to become knowledgeable in hair replacements. As the hair loss is greater, you'll need other options of servicing this client and that option will be another type of addition.

Comments

You will have clients who are very embarassed about their hair loss. You may want to consider designing an area in your salon where you can do hair addition services in private, out of sight from anyone else in the salon. Try not to make a "big deal" out of it. But, a private office for your consultation with clients and for those who want privacy during service is important. You may not be able to make the change in your salon right this minute. Keep it in mind for the future. And, always, remember a number of your clients and potential clients are embarassed. Be sensitive to their needs. If you can have a private room, consider booking these clients "after hours."

PLACEMENT PATTERN WORK SHEET for RAMIN

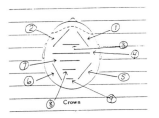

Track #	Attachment Method	Length of Hair	Color of Hair	Cost per in.	Width of Track	Times Density	= Total # of inches	Price for Hair	Estimate # of Hours	Perm Price per in.
1	Bond	8"	50		4"		4"			
2					4"		4"			
3					3"		3"			
4					5"		5"			
5					4"		4"			
6					4"		4"			
7					3"		3"			
8					2"		2"			
9	↓	↓	↓		1"		1"		↓	
TOTALS							30		1 hr	

JENNIFER – stylist: Douglas Kovalcik

Background Information and Services to Jennifer's Hair

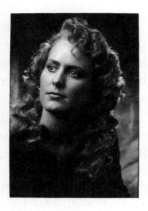

In case you can't guess, Jennifer is Arlene's daughter. The same hair type was passed on – that baby-fine hair. Jennifer, being younger and always ready to experiment, had really damaged her hair. The before picture doesn't show how green her hair was – but take my word for it. It was damaged, green hair!

Probably more times than not, a stylist who specializes in hair extensions must be a specialist in correction work. Clients who want and need hair extensions have one of two characteristics in common. They have problem hair (or hair problems) and they may experiment with anything to solve their problems, often causing more problems.

Because of the number of chemical services already done to Jennifer's own hair – perm-on-perm, color, highlighting, lowlighting and re-highlighting, corrective work was really required. Because she was already over-permed, we did not perm her hair. The color correction work involved removing the greenish cast by doing a "bleach wash" then, with a semi-permanent color, we made her a one-color blonde. As with Marla's hair, we used semi-permanent color. We plan to work with her hair care and color needs in the future and using semi-permanent color is less damaging than color requiring peroxide. The chemical services done to her hair should be reduced.

Services to Wefts

Because of time (too much to do in too short of a time) we decided to leave the wefts straight for this shoot. The wefts could have been permed, or we could have used factory permed hair.

We selected stage 8 (yellow orange) wefts that were a perfect match to Jennifer's new color, so no color work was necessary on the wefts.

Placement Pattern, etc.

Four tracks were put in her hair. Tracks #1 and #2 were double density of 16" hair. Track #3, also double density, was done with two different lengths of hair, 16" on the bottom and 12" on the top. The last track, #4 was single density of 8" hair. The total amount of hair used (by width of weft) was 68". Attachment time was approximately 4 hours.

CASE STUDIES

Finish/Styling

Jennifer's hair was set with a curling iron. As you can see, since the tracks are hidden, she can wear her hair down for her everyday style, up in a ponytail or up in an evening style.

Optional Approaches

Because of the condition of her own hair, the micro filler fiber braid was the best technique to use to hold and to protect her own hair.

Comments

Young clients who are interested in constant change and what I call the fast-food-syndrome approach to life do not make the best hair extension clients. There is a lot of time and money involved in hair extension services. Yet, there are people who are willing to pay for the "change" they want "now." You can service them, but know going in that this could be a very frustrating relationship. You are not your client's parent, you can't nag them. You are their professional consultant. We *all* do things we shouldn't. This is OK as long as we are willing to pay the price. By this I mean, as long as your clients are willing to recognize their responsibility and if they don't do the things they should, it still is their responsibility. You can fix it – but it will cost. I know clients who just can't be bothered to condition their hair properly or go to bed with wet hair. Well, it's OK, as long as they realize they'll need new hair more often and they'll need to come in for servicing more frequently.

PLACEMENT PATTERN WORK SHEET for JENNIFER

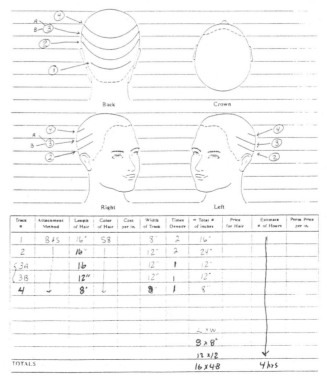

Track #	Attachment Method	Length of Hair	Color of Hair	Cost per in.	Width of Track	Times Density	= Total # of inches	Price for Hair	Estimate # of Hours	Perm Price per in.
1	B&S	16"	S8		8"	2	16"			
2		16"			12"	2	24"			
3A		16			12"	1	12"			
3B		12"			12"	1	12"			
4		8"			8"	1	8"			
							L x W			
							8 x 8"			
							12 x 12			
TOTALS							16 x 48		4 hrs	

ALONDRA – stylist: Douglas Kovalcik

Background Information and Services to Alondra's Hair

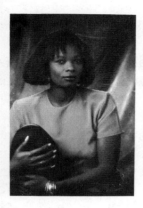

Alondra is a hairsylist and has been wearing hair extensions for many years. With her structure and her facal shape, etc., she can wear a *lot* of different styles. However, as a new owner of her own salon, life is very busy, so an easy-to-maintain style is best for her right now.

Unfortunately, Alondra was relaxing her own hair with her extensions in. As a result, she did severe damage to her own hair.

Prior to attaching the hair extensions, shampooing and conditioning were required for Alondra's hair.

Services to Wefts

The natural (brownish-black) color of Chinese or Indian hair is a good color for her. In this case we used factory permed hair that had a texture similar to extremely curly hair that has been relaxed.

Placement Pattern, etc.

The attachment technique was done with two micro filler fiber braided tracks. Tracks #1 and #2 were done with 12" hair, double density. The total amount of hair used was 48". The time required for attachment was approximately 2 hours.

Finish/Styling

With this style, Alondra's own hair was included in the front of the style. The extended hair was razor cut and the complete style was cut with scissors in a bob form, shorter in the nape area and in a curved formation which cupped into the back area (where she has a great deal of hair loss). The style then became longer, designed to swing toward her jawline.

The style was blown dry. Using a flat iron, it was finished off to give the hair a smoother texture. A styling gel was used to add sheen to the hair.

Optional Approaches

This style could also be created with total coverage, using the technique shown in Leann's style. In the case of total coverage, it doesn't make any difference what color hair is used. Also, the texture of the hair can be any texture desired. You could use hair that is factory permed, or hair that you perm to any curl desired, or even straight hair.

CASE STUDIES

Comments

One of the changes hair extensions are bringing about is a different approach to changing hair texture. For people with baby-fine hair, thick curly or wavy hair is now possible. No more frog-fuzz, frizzy impossible-to-manage-at-home hair! For people with extremely curly hair, no more constant harsh, damaging chemicals. They too can have silky, long, smooth, soft curls or waves or curls down their back. Just because your client's hair texture may end up "kinky" after chemical services does not mean they must have that texture. You can match it or change it. You can give them whatever they want in volume, length, color and texture.

PLACEMENT PATTERN WORK SHEET for ALONDRA

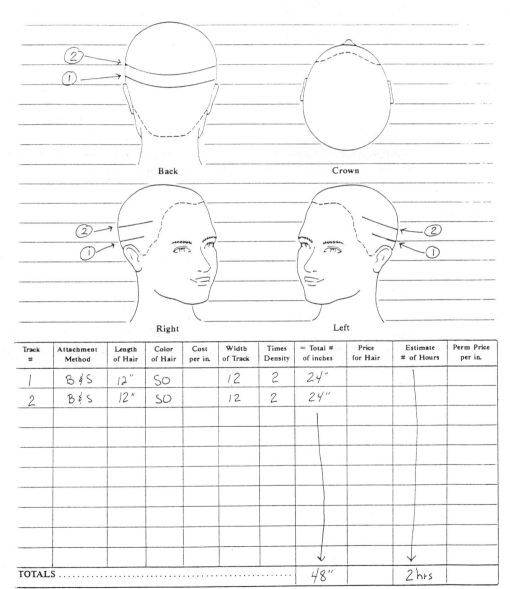

Track #	Attachment Method	Length of Hair	Color of Hair	Cost per in.	Width of Track	Times Density	= Total # of inches	Price for Hair	Estimate # of Hours	Perm Price per in.
1	B & S	12"	SO		12	2	24"			
2	B & S	12"	SO		12	2	24"			
TOTALS							48"		2 hrs	

CANDIDA – stylist: James Cristopher Chan

Background Information and Services to Candida's Hair

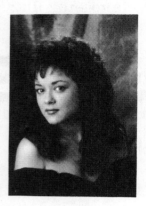

Candida used to have long hair and was sorry that she had it cut. So her reason for hair extensions is to have the look she loves back while she is waiting for her hair to grow out.

At only 18 years of age, Candida is working full time as a security guard with the goal of becoming a police officer. We all had to feel sorry for her because she had to work a full shift at night and then a long day for her hairstyling and the photo shoot.

She has a natural curl to her own hair with some color that was beginning to grow out. All that was needed was to do a soap cap to remove some of the red from her ends. (The soap cap is done by mixing equal parts of shampoo and 20 volume peroxide. This mixture is worked into the client's hair and left on for 5 to 10 minutes.)

Services to Wefts

Stage 1 (dark brown) wefts were custom permed with 9/16" rods (purple) to create the body wave. The reason for this type of curl was so it would have a wave but could also be blown dry for a smoother look.

Placement Pattern, etc.

There were five micro filler fiber braided tracks put in her hair, virtually complete coverage. In this situation, the placement pattern was designed to hide her own hair because it was so short and could not be blended in for an undetectable style.

Tracks #1 and #2 were done with double density 12" hair. Tracks #3, #4 and #5 were done with 8" hair, single density. The total amount of hair used was 67". The time required for tracking was 4 hours.

Finish/Styling

For a long, smooth style, Candida's hair was simply blown dry and brushed. As you can see, from short hair to long hair – in one day.

Because her tracking is well hidden, she can wear her hair in a very glamorous upsweep.

Optional Approaches

The bonding technique restricts some styling capabilities. The upsweep style would be difficult to accomplish if the wefts were bonded because bonded wefts do not pivot at the point of attachment as well as braided tracks or individual braids.

Both the down and upsweep styles can also be accomplished with individual braids. Attachment time required would be 10 to 15 hours.

Comments

The clients who can't wait for their hair to grow out are excellent hair extension prospects. Or even better, those whose hair just won't grow as long as they would like. A word of warning: hair longer than 16" is difficult for anyone to manage at home, particularly if you have never had long hair. As the hair is growing, the person gets used to taking care of long hair – all those little things you have to do to keep the tangles out. If a person's hair is naturally curly, they too are used to combing out the tangles. But if overnight a person has long hair – they usually don't know what to do with it. Let alone, if this person also acquires long, curly hair overnight – you and the client are probably going to have problems.

Another thing to remember, even if the client has had long hair and knows how to "live" with it, hair that is not growing from their scalp does not get the natural oils needed. Added hair requires a LOT of conditioning and extra care.

PLACEMENT PATTERN WORK SHEET for CANDIDA

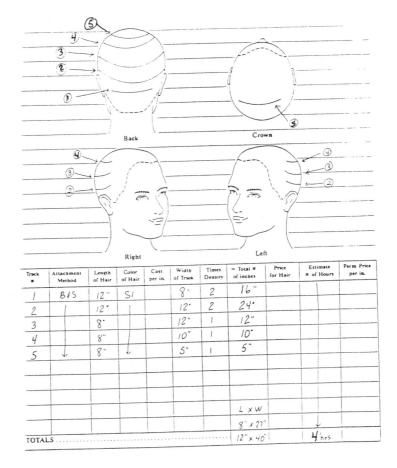

Track #	Attachment Method	Length of Hair	Color of Hair	Cost per in.	Width of Track	Times Density	= Total = of inches	Price for Hair	Estimate = of Hours	Perm Price per in.
1	B&S	12"	S1		8"	2	16"			
2		12"			12"	2	24"			
3		8"			12"	1	12"			
4		8"			10"	1	10"			
5	↓	8"	↓		5"	1	5"			
							L x W			
							8" x 27"			
TOTALS							12" x 40"		4 hrs	

JANICE – stylist: Lee Anthony

Background Information and Services to Janice's Hair

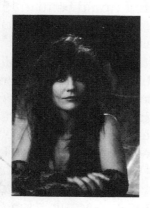

Janice, as a woman who is involved in sales, needs to look her best all the time. She does not have hair that allows the fullness needed to maintain a style. The hair added has given Janice's own hair not only fullness but a little additional length.

She is thin, of medium build. The ends of her hair had lightened to a reddish brown.

So that everything would blend together – we had to do a foil weave using a 3 level red-brown with 20 volume peroxide.

Services to Wefts

Actually, since we selected two different color wefts, a brownish-black (stage 0) and a dark brown (stage 1), we only had to shampoo and condition the wefts. No chemical services were required.

Placement Pattern, etc.

There were three braided tracks placed in Janice's hair. Tracks #1 and #2 were double density using 16" hair. The bottom weft was black and the top weft was dark brown. Track #3 was done with 12" hair, black on the bottom and dark brown on top. The total amount of hair used was 64". The approximate time required for this attachment was 3 hours.

Finish/Styling

After the wefts were sewn in, Janice's hair was razor cut together with the wefts to blend the hair together. She was given a root lift, which is done by taking large sections of hair, twisting them around your finger and clipping them only at the roots. Next you spray a setting lotion on the hair, dry it, remove the clips and rough up the hair a little. Voila – longer fuller hairstyle!

Optional Approaches

This style is also very appropriate for the individual braiding technique. The estimated time required would be 8 to 10 hours.

And, don't forget, this style can be accomplished by the addition of a fall. For clients with really active life styles, limited budgets, limited time – a 100% human hair fall may be the perfect answer. So, don't limit your thinking to only hair extension services. Remember – *The Fourth Dimension* means adding hair.

CASE STUDIES

Comments

Janice was wearing hair extensions when she came for her interview. And everyone could tell she was wearing extensions! You will get clients who have decided to come to you instead of going back to the stylist that did their extension service before. Be sure to ask why they are coming to you. Naturally, if they've moved or for other reasons their stylist is no longer available, it's easy – you are able to immediately start with a "clean slate." However, if they are the kind of client who will not take responsibility for the care of their own hair and want to blame someone else – be forewarned. If the service they received was not good or not professional – remember diplomacy. Don't ever put-down another stylist. Be positive with the client, be informative, let the client know how knowledgeable you are by doing a thorough complete consultation.

PLACEMENT PATTERN WORK SHEET for JANICE

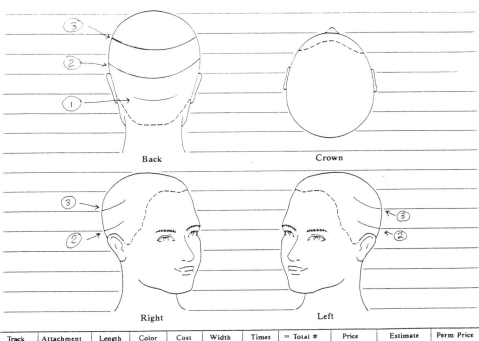

Track #	Attachment Method	Length of Hair	Color of Hair	Cost per in.	Width of Track	Times Density	= Total # of inches	Price for Hair	Estimate # of Hours	Perm Price per in.
1A	B&S	16"	SO		8"	1	8"			
1B		16"	S1		8"	1	8"			
2A		16"	SO		12"	1	12"			
2B		16"	S1		12"	1	12"			
3A		12"	SO		12"	1	12"			
3B	↓	12"	S1		12"	1	12"			
							L × W			
							12" × 12" — SO			
							16" × 18" — SO			
							12" × 12" — S1	↓		
TOTALS							16" × 18" — S1	3 hrs.		

SUSAN – stylist: James Cristopher Chan

Background Information and Services to Susan's Hair

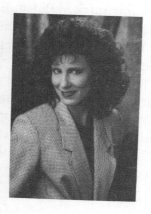

Susan is another example of what The Fourth Dimension is all about! Susan is an interior decorator in southern California. As a professional woman, her life is busy, but she needs "the look." She has very fine hair and has had a lot of problems with breakage from perms. She lives at the beach so her hair is constantly subjected to the elements. She does not like one bit of red in her hair so she over-shampoos and colors it, causing more damage.

Susan was given a partial perm on the top and sides. The color build-up was lifted during the perming process. Her hair was also conditioned.

Services to Wefts

Dark brown (stage 1) wefts were a perfect match so no coloring was required. They were custom permed to match Susan's permed curl.

Placement Pattern, etc.

There were 5 micro filler fiber braids tracked in Susan's own hair. Track #1 and #2 were double density using 8" hair. Tracks #3 and #4 were done single density with 12" hair. Track #5 was single density of 8" hair. The total amount of hair used was 69". The time required for attachment was approximately 4 hours.

Finish/Styling

After attachment, the wefts were razor cut and the style was cut in with shears. Her hair was diffuser-dried. Gel and mousse were used for the finish.

Optional Approaches

This style can also be accomplished using the individual braiding technique. However, it would not be advisable until the stylist and the client have spent more time together. A client with hair extensions should not do home chemical services to their own hair. The client will need to adjust to totally trusting the stylist and must schedule more time and money for hair care.

Also, remember, this is a client who wanted *long* hair. After a month or two, if the client has successfully managed their hair extensions, you may want to go ahead and give the client the longer hair desired.

Another approach for this type of client would be to consider a fall. This would give this client the look desired with less maintenance problems.

CASE STUDIES

Comments

Susan is another perfect type of hair extension client. She was ready for a change in her life – and that even meant a new look. She was willing to learn new hair care habits. Her hair will be always at odds with the elements. The beach and the sun will continue to change her color, but as a stylist you can help this kind of client to maintain the desired look.

PLACEMENT PATTERN WORK SHEET for SUSAN

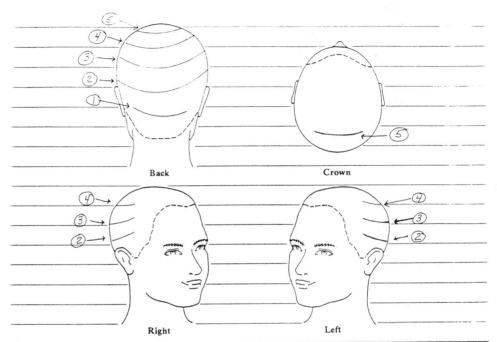

Track #	Attachment Method	Length of Hair	Color of Hair	Cost per in.	Width of Track	Times Density	= Total # of inches	Price for Hair	Estimate # of Hours	Perm Price per in.
1	B&S	8"	S1		8"	2	16"			
2		8"			12"	2	24"			
3		12"			12"	1	12"			
4		12"			12"	1	12"			
5	↓	8"	↓		5"	1	5"			
								L × W		
								8" × 45"	↓	
TOTALS							12" × 24"	4 hrs.		

LYNN – stylist: Lee Anthony

Background Information and Services

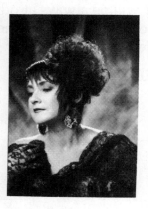

Hairstylists are customers too! Lynn has been a stylist for a number of years and was interested in a fun look.

Lynn's hair was simply shampooed and conditioned.

The wefts were custom permed. Some were permed with a tight curl, others were done with a looser curl. This is a fun style you can do using "scraps" of your leftover wefts. We used 8" wefts in four different colors, stages 0, 1, 2 and 8 – brownish black, dark brown, reddish brown, yellow orange. Some wefts were colored different shades of red. One was made a burgundy color.

Placement Pattern, etc.

A circular pattern was braided in the crown area. The wefts were sewn in, mixing the different colors together. The weft on the side was bonded. The approximate amount of hair used was 51". The attachment time was approximately 2 hours.

Finish/Styling

This style is a combination of hair added by tracking on the top of her head, and then on the sides, red and black hair was bonded in. The hair was razor cut, blown dry. Then taking a razor, the hair was fringed toward her face.

Optional Approaches

Because this was a fun style, the attachment techniques could be anything you wanted. Micro filler fiber braids and bonding were used. Naturally you could also do individual braids.

Another alternative would be to use a wiglet, curling and coloring it to make your "creation."

Comments

This style is fun – to create, to cut, to style, to wear! Remember the other people who work in your salon. Do something different, something exciting on their hair. It's practice for you, fun for them and advertising for you.

This is a great look for that big event. Your imagination is your only limitation when it comes to hair extension services and styles!

CASE STUDIES

PLACEMENT PATTERN WORK SHEET for LYNN

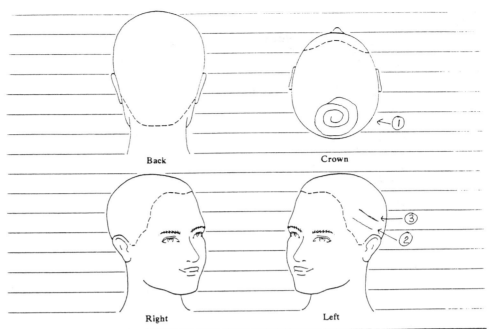

Back　　　　　　　　Crown

Right　　　　　　　　Left

Track #	Attachment Method	Length of Hair	Color of Hair	Cost per in.	Width of Track	Times Density	= Total # of inches	Price for Hair	Estimate # of Hours	Perm Price per in.
1	B&S	8"	*				45"			
2	Bond	8"	S-0				3"			
3	Bond	8"	S-0				3"			
	* mix	of S0, S1, S2 & S8								
							L x W		↓	
TOTALS							8" x 51"		2 hrs	

KATHLEEN – Stylist: Lee Anthony

Background Information and Services to Kathleen's Hair

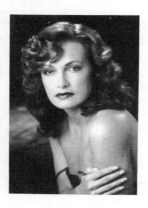

Kathleen is also a hairstylist. She has fine textured hair and wanted extensions to create more volume and hair color depth.

Her hair was three dimensionally colored. Three different levels of red were created by using different volumes of peroxide. In the nape area, level 3 color with 10 volume peroxide was processed for 30 minutes. Just above the occipital bone and below the crown in the front to the temple area above the ears, level 4 color with 20 volume peroxide was processed for 30 minutes. The third level of red was in the crown area to the front hairline. This color was created using level 5 color with 40 volume peroxide; processing time was 15 minutes.

Service to Wefts

In this case we used 12" natural black wefts. They were custom permed using 9/16" (purple) rods in a spiral wrap. An alkaline perm was used. Following the perm the wefts were lightened using 20 volume peroxide with powder bleach for 10 minutes. Then the wefts were colored with a level 4 red using 20 volume peroxide for 30 minutes.

Placement Pattern, etc.

There were two tracks braided to create this style. Tracks #1 and #2 were double density. A total of 38" of hair was used. Attachment time was approximately 2 hours.

Finish/Styling

Kathleen's hair was razor and scissor cut. Her finished style was done with a pin curl and roller set which was just brushed out into waves to create the pageboy style.

To add to the beauty of this style is the depth of color. As explained above, there were three dimensions of color in Kathleen's own hair – then a fourth dimension was added with the fourth color of the wefts.

Optional Approaches

Bonding would be an acceptable attachment technique, if you did not put the style up since bonding does restrict the movement of the hair. Individual braiding could also be used to accomplish this style.

CASE STUDIES

Comments

Hair extensions are a wonderful way to add volume to anyone who needs it. With clients with really nice hair – but of a fine texture, the adding of volume allows styling capabilities not possible before. The style will last longer. While you're at it – add some fun, add color excitement.

PLACEMENT PATTERN WORK SHEET for KATHLEEN

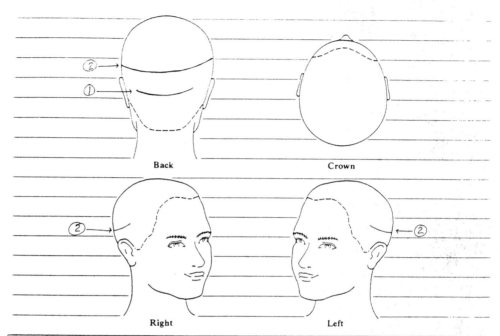

Track #	Attachment Method	Length of Hair	Color of Hair	Cost per in.	Width of Track	Times Density	= Total # of inches	Price for Hair	Estimate # of Hours	Perm Price per in.
1	B & S	12"			7"	2	14"			
2	B & S	12"			12"	2	24"			
TOTALS							38"		2 hrs	

ERIN – Stylist: Lee Anthony

Background Information and Services to Erin's Hair and Wefts

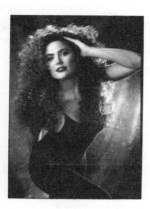

Erin has naturally naturally curly hair with many types of texture throughout. She is a professional model. Because she is tall, she can carry off 24" hair.

Her hair was foil weaved to lighten the dark hair around her face to match the sun-streaked hair further out.

We used three different color wefts: stage 1 (dark brown) stage 3 (reddish brown) and stage 8 (yellow orange). No additional coloring was required.

To match the many textures of Erin's own hair we used several textures of hair. Some of the hair was factory permed and some of the hair was custom permed.

Placement Pattern, etc.

There were three tracks done on this style. Track #1 was double density of 24" hair. On track #2, on the bottom of the track 24" hair was placed and on the top, 20" hair. On track #3 all the hair was 20", double density. The total number of inches used was 42". Total attachment time required was 3 hours.

Finish/Styling

Erin's hair was dried, then set with a device called wave conductors, which created a very spiral look to her hair.

Then, for the next shots, we used pomade to open up the curls, creating a fuller look.

Remember, this style is very limited. This amount of hair requires a lot of work to maintain. But, for clients who want long hair – here it is!

Optional Approaches

This style could also be created by using the individual braiding technique. However, this is really too much hair for almost anyone to be able to manage. I know a number of stylists who have clients who are dancers and need long hair that moves with them – so extensions are the answer. However, this much hair is almost impossible to dry, or comb out, or manage on your own. So an alternative attachment method is to make micro filler fiber braided tracks. Then sew clips on to the wefts. This way the clients can put on their wefts before they go onstage but remove them otherwise. They don't have to shampoo them, sleep with them and deal with that much hair all the time.

CASE STUDIES

Comments

It's show time! This much hair is not for most people. But it is appropriate for show business.

For dancers, singers, musicians, people who have professions that require the *"bigger than life"* image – hair extensions can be the answer.

PLACEMENT PATTERN WORK SHEET for ERIN

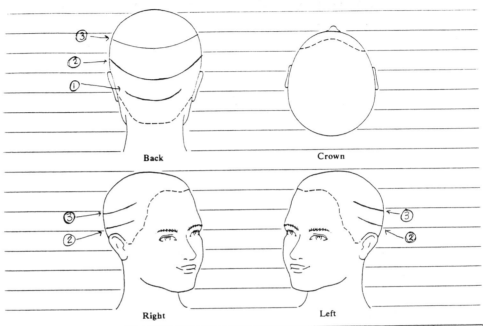

Back · Crown · Right · Left

Track #	Attachment Method	Length of Hair	Color of Hair	Cost per in.	Width of Track	Times Density	= Total # of inches	Price for Hair	Estimate # of Hours	Perm Price per in.
1	B & S	24"	S1		8"	2	16"			
2A	↓	24"	S3		12"	1	12"			
2B		20"	S8		12"	1	12"			
3A		20"	S3		12"	1	12"			
3B	↓	20"	S8		12"	1	12"			
							L x W — Color			
							24" x 16' — S1			
							24" x 12 — S3			
							20" x 12 — S3			
TOTALS							20" x 24 — S8			

GENERAL COMMENTS

Remember the things that infleunce your decisions about accepting and servicing hair extension clients. The questions you'll ask yourself are:

- if you want this client
- if the client's hair is in acceptable condition
- if the client has enough hair for attachment
- if the tracking hair can be hidden

Use your consultation form to better understand your future client:

- reason for extensions
- life style (work and recreation)
- home care habits
- salon habits
- hair condition
- scalp condition
- stature, face and head shape
- sensitivities to products
- growth patterns particularly areas of baldness

With the proper information, you can *create a miracle*. You can make a difference for many people.

Chapter 10

MARKETING AND SALES

INTRODUCTION

The terms marketing and sales have to do with presenting and selling your products and services.

Marketing primarily means the method of presenting your products and services to the public.

Sales means making the actual sale to a specific client.

ADVERTISING

There are many ways to advertise your services.

Bold type in the white pages of the telephone book
Ads in the yellow pages
Newspaper advertising
Flyers and Brochures

These all are all ways of telling your story. However all of these things cost money and to begin with, I'd like to suggest that you use the PR (Public Relations) approach.

PUBLIC RELATIONS

First, it is always a good idea to try out your skills on co-workers, friends and family members. They will allow you to practice and to learn.

They are available so that you can observe what kinds of problems may develop. Then you can figure out how to eliminate or deal with these problems before you have a paying client. (Be sure to charge your co-workers/friends/family members for the hair and any other out-of-pocket expenses. There should be *some* investment on their part too!)

Then, when you are ready, contact your local newspaper.

Sample Press Release

This is a sample press release to send to various media with before and after photos.

Be sure to **double-space** the press release.

```
CONTACT
Your Name
Salon/School Name
Salon/School Address
City, State, Zip
Phone (    )

FOR IMMEDIATE RELEASE
Month & Year


HUMAN HAIR EXTENSIONS REVOLUTIONIZE SALON SERVICES
(your City, State) --- Human hair extensions, the
revolutionary Fourth Dimension in professional salon
services, are available at (Salon/school Name, Phone
(   )      , Street Address, City).

The professionals at (Salon/School Name) customize
the color, texture and length of 100% human hair wefts
to a perfect match with your own hair. You can achieve
a total fashion transformation with all-natural ex-
tensions that are virtually undetectable.

Human hair extensions may be attached by any of several
safe techniques. For example, your stylist might
create micro-braids in your hair and sew the wefts
onto those braided tracks. Wefts can also be attached
to your hair with a latex-based adhesive. Safe at-
tachment methods such as these will maintain the
health and condition of your own hair while you enjoy
your extensions style. Depending upon the rate at
which your hair grows, the wefts will be reattached
after about four to eight weeks.

Call (your phone #) today for a consultation.
```

MARKETING AND SALES

Sample Editorial Write-up

```
HUMAN HAIR EXTENSIONS:
THE FOURTH DIMENSION OF HAIR DESIGN
```

Human Hair Extensions, the revolutionary Fourth Dimension of Hair Design, put instant length and volume into the hands of the professional hairstylist.

"Until now, we were limited to working with the client's existing hair in our attempts to achieve the best possible look for them," says (stylist's name), professional hairstylist since (date).

"Human hair extensions utilize all of the stylist's skills in perming, coloring and cutting hair -- the first three dimensions of hair design."

Whether you have baby-fine hair and have dreamed of more hair all your life, or your hair has thinned over the years and you want thicker hair that will make you look 20 years younger, human hair extensions are the answer to your prayers.

"The best reward we receive by doing hair extensions is the way people react when we're done," explains (name of salon owner), owner of (salon name). "They exhibit such an increase in self-confidence when they look in the mirror and they always express a more positive outlook on life."

If you have admired long hair and your own hair is simply too short, hair extensions offer the instant solution. Maybe you have wanted a thick, fuller style and you already have enough length, extensions can be added for volume only.

"The transformation from 'Before' to 'After' human hair extensions is amazing," (stylist's name) says. "The human hair wefts are customized to match the client's own hair color and texture. This makes them virtually undetectable and the finished hairstyle looks absolutely natural."

Human hair extensions may be attached by any of several safe techniques. For example, your stylist might create micro-braids in your hair and sew the hair wefts onto those braided tracks. Wefts can also be attached to your hair with a latex-based adhesive. Safe attachment methods such as these will maintain the health and condition of your own hair while you experience the luxury of an excellent style created just for you.

Depending upon the rate at which your hair grows, the hair wefts will be reattached after about four to eight weeks.

Sample Letter to Editors:

You might choose to notify your local beauty/fashion editors and writers about human hair extension services and education. A letter such as this and a hand written invitation (gift certificate for hair extensions) could lead to editorial coverage of your business.

```
DATE

MAGAZINE OR NEWSPAPER
ATTENTION: BEAUTY AND/OR FASHION EDITOR
ADDRESS
CITY, STATE, ZIP



Dear (name):

Human hair extensions are revolutionizing the profes-
sional salon industry. In addition to the existing
cut, perm and color options, human hair extensions
represent an exciting Fourth Dimension.

At (your school/salon name), we are highly skilled in
the design and safe attachment methods for 100% human
hair extensions.

In sharp contrast with synthetic fiber (plastic) ex-
tensions, human hair is completely natural. 100% human
hair wefts may be permed and/or colored to a perfect
match with the client's own hair. The wefts are avail-
able in five lengths -- from 8" to a waist-length 24".

The before-and-after transformations are striking.
The stylist customizes each extensions service to suit
the individual's specific beauty needs and budget
parameters.

As an introduction to this revolutionary new service,
(individual's name(s) and title(s) here) invites you
to visit our school/salon for a complimentary human
hair extension style for you or a friend.

Please feel free to contact me for more information
and photos. I look forward to your call.

Sincerely,

(YOUR NAME and
TELEPHONE NUMBER)
```

COMMUNITY ACTIVITIES

Every stylist I know doing hair extension services says that a majority of their business comes by word-of-mouth. Satisfied clients, although they won't tell *everyone,* will tell their families and best friends. Your own work is always your best advertisement. And, if you think of every style you do as a walking advertisement, you'll get a lot of business.

However, there are many ways you can develop business by being active in your community. You can do volunteer work at hospitals, for fashion shows, and fund-raising events. In all kinds of community activities you can meet people and share your expertise with them.

You can also join a speakers bureau. Give talks before clubs within your community. "Whoa, hold it a minute!" you say. "Me, a public speaker?" Well, isn't that part of your job? Isn't that what you do everyday when you talk to a client? When you answer the telephone?

Here is where I'd like to give you a strong suggestion. I'd like to suggest you spend two hours a week improving your communications skills – and having fun while you do it! The way you can do this is to join a local Toastmasters International Program. There are thousands of clubs all over the world. Send for a free brochure by writing to:

Toastmasters International Program
2200 North Grand Avenue
PO Box 10400
Santa Ana, CA 92711, USA
Telephone: 714/542-6793 Fax: 714/543-7801

I could go on and on about Toastmasters and how it has helped me and so many people I know. Give it a try.

IN-SALON SALES

Telephone Inquiries

You know how people will call and ask prices of your services. Well, with hair extension services – it's even more of a problem. It is impossible to give any information on the telephone. So you have to get the prospective client to come in first. With someone who's never been to your salon, you will need to do a sales job to book the consultation. Then, the consultation is a form of sales for the service.

NEVER give prices on the telephone! It is necessary to book a consultation appointment first. To do this, the client may want to come in to see what you do and what can be done. Book a *presentation appointment* with the receptionist or the stylist.

Point-of-Purchase Sales

Now, you have a prospective client in your salon. Your receptionist can have the responsibility of making the "close" for the consultation appointment. Remember, the consultation requires the stylist's **time** and time is money. That is why a fee should be charged for the consultation. Such a fee also makes the client aware, right in the beginning, of the value of hair extension services.

To help the prospective client understand the services provided, you can have a number of tools to assist you.

Create a brochure that explains the services. Show the prospect a book with before-and-after pictures. By the way, if you do before-and-after pictures of your clients, be sure to have them sign a release form. (See Chapter 8.) If the stylist doing the hair extension services has attended a course – display the certificate.

If you have a video player at the salon, show videos created just for this purpose – consumer education/sales.

Another helpful tool is the Manikin. You can have Manikins done with the various attachment techniques that you use. Letting the client see and touch the micro filler fiber braids, individual braids or bonded tracks can help them understand exactly what is involved.

A NEW LIFE – A NEW DIMENSION

Hair extension services can be, literally, a new life or a new lease on life for you. If you are reaching "stylist burn out" – if you feel that it's just a job and your work has lost the excitement and fun you first knew – look to *The Fourth Dimension*.

If you are interested in continuing to be in the forefront of our industry – look to the new dimension – *The Fourth Dimension*.

If you have moved and have not built up a clientele or are new to our industry and don't have a clientele – what better way to build one? Become an expert, a specialist in adding hair.

Join me in – *The Fourth Dimension!*

INDEX

A

Accepting client 248
Accommodate your client 225
Add-ons definition 2
Additions serve four purposes 2
Additions three categories 2
Adhesive bond 127
Advantages/disadvantages
    braiding and sewing 26
    bonding 128
    individual braiding techniques 90
Advertising 242, 249
Analysis pre-color 155
Analysis pre-perm 140
Anthony, Lee styles by
  . . . . 212, 213, 222, 230, 238, 242, 244, 246
Areas of scalp to avoid 79
Attaching wefts 83, 129
Attachment techniques definitions . . . 11, 20-23

B

Baldness/balding 70, 79, 87, 126, 135, 231
Best technique 23
Bleach wash 218, 232
Bleached hair (see decolorization)
Blood pressure down, new hairstyle 1
Blotting perm 147, 148
Bond
    applying 131, 132
    removing 133-135
    test strip 135
    understanding 136
    techniques 11, 21, 127-136
Braid
    definition 9
    too tight 79
Braid-in tie-off with
    loose hair, individual braiding 110-121
    thread, individual braiding 122, 123
Braided support finish of tracks 82, 87
Braiding
    four types for tracks 25
    individual techniques 89-126
    practice 25, 27
    tracks 21, 25-88
Brick-layer pattern
for individual braids 93, 111, 124, 125
Brush-back placement pattern 169
Bulk hair 17, 91
Burn test for hair 12

C

Cabling tracks 22
Case studies 211-226
    Alondra 234
    Arlene 226
    Candida 236
    Dana 216
    Erin 246
    Janice 238
    Jennifer 232
    Kathleen 244
    Larry 220
    Leann 218
    Lynn 242
    Marla 228
    Monnique 214
    Ramin 230
    Susan 240
    Wanda 222
    Zettoria 224
Chan, James Cristopher
styles by 212, 224, 236, 240
Changing stylists 215, 239
Chemical service record (figure 12) 204
Chemical services release (figure 8) 199
China hair from 11
Chrome dyed hair 16, 139
Circular placement patterns 167, 168
Clean braids 69
Client
    comfort 219
    head regarding perming wefts 143
    new 215, 239
    public image 1, 217, 246
    hair captured in bond 135
    hair captured in braid 88
Clothes and shoes for comfort 35
Collecting and grading hair 14
Color
    client's hair 186
    coverage 159
    custom 151-162
    lowlighting or highlighting 159, 160
    mix-match 161, 238
    original hair 11, 16, 152
    product selection 155
    rules 156
    test for hair 13
    test strand 159
Colored at factory 16, 153
Coloring
    hair extensions 151-162
    hair that cannot/should not be 154
Colors of synthetic fibers 19
Combinations placement patterns 172
Community activities 253
Condition of client's hair 184
Consultation
    chemical service record 204
    chemical services release 199
    hair costing sheet 196
    hair extension agreement 200
    hair extension release 203
    hair pricing sheet 198
    home care instructions 205-210
    model's agreement/release 202

objectives 180
services price sheet 194
work sheet 181-194
work sheet (figure 1) 182
work sheet (figure 2) 187
work sheet (figure 3) 190
work sheet (figure 4) 192
Control fingers 35, 41, 42, 51, 60, 71, 92, 110
Cortex definition 4
Cortex porosity 140
Cotton covered polyester thread 28, 82, 83
Cramping from braiding 29, 35, 80, 88
Cross sections synthetic fibers 19
Curling and finishing style 174
Curvature of head 80
Custom coloring hair 153
Cut hair (root turned) 13
Cut
layering angles 173
razor 172, 173
style 172
Cuticle
definition 4
porosity 139
scrubbing 16
stripped 13, 15, 16

D

Decisions about accepting client 248
Decolorization 11, 16, 152, 153, 158
Density
client's hair 185
hair of individual braid 124
hair of weft 141
Design (see placement pattern)
Design variations 164
Designing and styling techniques 163-174
Diameters synthetic fibers 19
Double density weft attachment 83-88
Double-density wefts 18
Drawing cards 9
Dyed hair 16, 139, 153
Dyes chrome 16, 139, 153
Dyes progressive (see chrome dyes) 155

E

Editorial sample 251
Elasticity 141, 185
Europe hair from 11
European wavy 18
Exercises 28-34
Expert in coloring 161
Expert in perming 149
Extensions definition 2, 9
Extensions reason for 183

F

Facial shape 188
Factory colored hair 16, 139, 153
Factory permed hair 139
Facts about wefts, coloring 152
Facts about wefts, perming 138

Fashion Fun
asymmetrical 170
bangs 170
color accents 171
ponytail 169
volume 170
Fast-food-syndrome 233
Fifteen minutes perming 147, 148
Filler fiber 28, 42-50, 60-69, 70-79
Fine hair 219
Finger positions
braiding and sewing 35, 41, 42, 51, 60, 71
individual braiding 92, 110
Fingers
control 35, 41, 42, 51, 60, 71, 92, 110
working 35, 41, 42, 51, 60, 71, 92, 110
Finishing off tracks 81
Finishing the style 174
Foil coloring hair 160
Fold-over for individual braiding 93, 111, 122, 123
Fold-over weft hair 18
Form hair 185
Forms
chemical service record 204
chemical services release statement 199
consultation work sheet . . . 182, 187, 190, 192
hair costing sheet 196
hair extension agreement 200
hair extension release 203
hair pricing sheet 198
home care instructions 206
models agreement/release 202
sample services price sheet 195
Fourth dimension definition 2

G

Glue attachment 22
Gray hair 161
Growth patterns 186

H

Habits home care 183
Habits salon 184
Hackle .9
Hair
China 11
Europe 11
India 11
bulk 17
chrome dyed 16, 139
collecting and grading 14
colors 152, 186
condition 184
costing sheet 196
curl natural body 141
density 185
density and placement 124
differences 5
elasticity 185
extension agreement 200
extension release 203
factory permed 139
facts for coloring 152

Index 257

facts for perming 138-140
foil coloring 160
form 185
gray 161
growth preparations 230
labeling 12
layers 4
length 173, 185
loose 17
loss from extensions 70, 79, 87, 88, 126, 135, 231
lowlighting or highlighting 159
porosity 184
pre-color analysis 155
preparation for bonding 129
prepare for individual braiding 91
prepare for perming 144
pricing sheet 198
processing 15
testing 12
texture 184
that cannot/should not be colored . . . 154
that cannot/should not be permed . . . 139
uses 12
weighing, bundling and storing 14, 15
white 161
Hairpieces (see add-ons and replacements)
Hand barrier cream 92
Hand-tied weft 17, 18
Hands fingers and wrists
braiding and sewing . . . 35, 41, 42, 51, 60, 71
individual braiding 92, 110
Hands prepare for speed-bonding 92
Hazardous attachment 22, 23
Head shape 189
Heartbeat slowed, new hairstyle 1
Helix, double . . . . Preface, 50
Highlighting hair 159
Home care habits 183
Home care instructions 205-210
Hot spots 79, 80
Human hair information about 11
Human relations ten commandments 175

I

In-salon sales 253
India hair from 11
Individual braiding
definition 10, 17, 21
density 124
maintaining and re-doing 125, 126
pattern brick-layer 93, 111, 124, 125
technique, locking descriptions 89
technique, loose hair
braid-in tie-off 110-121
technique, separate tie-off 123, 124
technique, speed-bonding 89-126
technique, thread braid-in tie-off . . . 122, 123
Indonesian hair from 12
Interlock weaving 22
Interweaving techniques 17

K

Kovalcik, Douglas
styles by 212, 226, 228, 232, 234

L

Latex bond 127
Law of color 156, 157
Layering angles 173
Layers of hair 4
Length desired 185
Length perming weft 141
Letter to editor sample 252
Life style .183
Line of demarcation 172
Lock in twist 43, 72
Lock-stitch 82
Locking techniques
for individual braids 89
Long hair .237
Loose hair, bulk hair 17, 23, 91
Lowlighting or highlighting 159

M

Machine made wefts 17, 18
Maintaining and re-doing the style
bonding technique 133
braid and sew 88
individual braid technique 125, 126
Manikin
head 27
holder 27
set up for coloring 160
set up for individual braiding 91
set up for perming 144
set up, braiding and sewing 35
Marketing 249
Medically proved hairstyle improves health . . . 1
Medulla of hair shaft 4
Micro filler fiber braid 10, 70-82
Mix-match colors of wefts 161, 238
Modacrylic, synthetic fibers 19
Model's agreement/release form (figure 10) . .202
Movement of wrist . 35, 41, 42, 51, 60, 71, 92, 110
Muriatic acid 15
Music play for rhythm 35

N

Natural body 141
Needles for braid and sew technique 28, 83
Neutralizing muriatic acid 16
Neutralizing perm 148, 149
News release sample 250
Non-dyed hair 16
Nylon, synthetic fibers 19

O

Organizing time 178
Over braiding 89-126
Over-sewing 85

P

PEP USA 28
PVC, synthetic fibers 19
Pain 70, 80
Parkinson's Educational Program 28

Perm
- apply solution 146
- becoming an expert 149
- blotting 147, 148
- categories 142
- fifteen minute wait 147, 148
- hair extensions 137-150
- neutralizing 148
- no heat 146
- prepare the hair 144
- product selection 142
- rinse after neutralizing 149
- rinse after processing 147
- test 13
- test curls 146
- test strand 145
- wrap hair 145

Permanent color 155
Placement for individual braid technique . . . 124
Placement of filler fiber 43, 61, 62, 71, 72
Placement patterns (see design)
Placement pattern
- 2-tracks 81, 164, 214, 234, 244
- 3-tracks 165, 216, 224, 238, 246
- 4-tracks 167, 220, 228, 232
- 5-track 236, 240
- 6-tracks 166
- 7-tracks 230
- 8-tracks 222
- asymmetrical 170
- bangs 170
- brush-back/brush-up 169
- circular 167, 168, 169, 218, 242
- color accents 171
- combinations 172, 242
- fashion fun 169-171
- full coverage 166, 168, 218
- ponytail 169
- volume 170, 223, 226, 230, 240, 244

Plastic bag for perming 146
Polyester, synthetic fibers 19
Polypropylene, synthetic fibers 19
Ponytail finish of track 81, 86, 87
Ponytail placement pattern 169
PoPractice braiding on person's head 27
Pre-color analysis of hair 155
Pre-perm analysis 140
Prepare hair coloring 158
Prepare hair perming 144
Price sheet for service sample 195
Pricing work sheet 192
Problem hair 215, 219
Processed/processing hair 13, 15, 16
Porosity
- client's hair 184
- cortex 140
- cuticle 139
- weft 140, 155

Products sensitivity to 127, 186
Professional value 1
Professional women 223, 227, 241
Progressive dyes 155
Public relations 249

Pulling hair out from scalp 70, 87, 126, 135
Putting it all together 175

R

Race, hair has no 4, 221
Range of motion exercises 28-34
Rash on scalp 80
Razor cut 172, 173
Reason for extensions 183
Record keeping 178
Removing
- cuticle 13, 15, 16
- individual braids 125
- speed-bonding 125
- wefts 88

Replacements 2, 231
Responsible, How Am I 21, 24
Restructuring curl 220, 234
Rinsing neutralizer 149
Rinsing perm 147
Root perm 226
Root-turned hair 13
Rubber (latex) bond 127
Rubber bands 27
Rules color 156

S

Sales and marketing 249
Sales in-salon 253
Salon habits 184
Sample
- editorial 251
- letter to editor 252
- news release 250
- services price sheet 195

Scalp
- areas to avoid 79
- condition 185
- rash 80
- redness 79

Scrubbing cuticle 16
Securing ends of braid and sew tracks 86
Semi-permanent color 155
Sensitive scalp 79, 127
Sensitive to 127, 186
Separate tie-off individual braiding 123, 124
Services price sheet 191, 195
Sewing machines 17, 18
Sewing wefts to tracks 83-87
Sex, hair has no 4, 221
Shape facial 188
Shape head 189
Shears working 28
Shino, Keiko styles by . . . 213, 214, 216, 218, 220
Single density weft attachment 87
Single-density wefts 18
Soap cap 236
Speed-bond description 28
Speed-bond remover 125
Speed-bonding individual braid
lock-in technique 91-110
Speed-bonding thread when tracking . . . 86, 87

Stages of Lightening (see decolorization) . . . 152
Stature 184
Stitch lock 82
Storing hair .14
Stripping cuticle 13, 15, 16
Style curling and finishing 174
Style cutting 172
Styling techniques 163-174
Stylists for this book
   Lee Anthony
       . . . . . . .212, 213, 222,230, 238, 242, 244, 246
      James Cristopher Chan 212, 224, 236, 240
      Douglas Kovalcik 212, 226, 228, 232, 234
      Keiko Shino 213, 214, 216, 218, 220
Stylists as clients 242, 244
Stylists dealing with 215, 239
Sun effects 241, 246
Supplies
   bonding techniques 129
   braiding and sewing 26
   coloring hair extensions 152
   consultation 179
   designing and styling 163
   individual braiding 91
   perming hair extensions 138
Synthetic fibers 19, 20

T

T-pin weft to Manikin 145, 160
Teamwork 176,204
Techniques best 23
Techniques other 22
Temporary color 155
Ten commandments of human relations . . . 175
Tension on braids 36-80
Terms definition of 8
Test strand color 159
Test strand perm 145
Texture change 235
Texture weft 141, 155, 184
Thinning hair 230
Thread cotton covered polyester 28, 82, 83
Track design (see placement patterns)
Tracks
   braided 70-88
   definition 9
   finishing off 81, 82

U

Un-do braided tracks 88
Under braid 35-41
Under braid on scalp 51-59
Under filler fiber braid 42-50
Under filler fiber braid on scalp 60-80

W

Wax attachment 22
Weaving
   definition 11
   hair between threads 9
   machine .9
   making wefts 8
   poles 9
   thread tracks 22
Weft
   definition 9
   density 18, 141
   fold-over 18
   hair length 173
   hand-tied 9, 17, 18
   machine made 17, 18
   sewing to tracks 83-87
White hair 161
Working fingers . . . 35, 41, 42, 51, 60, 71, 92, 110
Wrapping techniques for perming wefts . . .143
Wrist movement . . . 35, 41, 42, 51, 60, 71, 92, 110